Marianne E. Meyer

SPIRULINA

Survival food for a new era

Delicious recipes with the primal nourishment

Amazing healing success with the blue-green alga

The information introduced in this book was carefully researched and imparted in all conscience. However, author and publisher do not take any liability for damages of any nature that could emerge directly or indirectly from the usage or application of the data in this book. The data of this work is for interested parties and education.

© 2016 by Marianne E. Meyer, Tavira, Portugal
All rights are with the author
drmarianneemeyer@gmail.com
www.marianne-e-meyer.com

Herstellung und Verlag:
BoD - Books on Demand, Norderstedt
ISBN 978-3-734728525

Photo credits:
Cover photo: *Fa. Cyanotech, Anissa Brauneis*
Cover back: Cyanotech ,
Inner part: R. Taylor 2, 17,29,36, 41,42,64,76,
Earthrise 36, Sanatur 41,74,84
Görke, J. 67,68, M. Zinn 79, C.-P. Meyer 83,
Cover, typography & typesetting: M. Meyer

Some other books by M. E. Meyer:

How Water Connects our Worlds
Doris Day and my Search for Relatives
Migrant Birds on Wheels
Spirulina, das blaugrüne Wunder
Cranberry Powerfrucht
Psyllium - So bekommen Sie Ihr Fett weg
Spirulina für Kinder

Marianne Meyer, Apartado 320
P-8801 Tavira

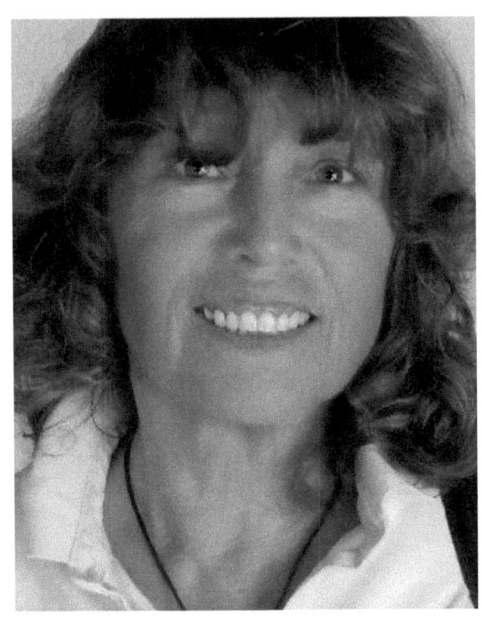

Marianne E. Meyer has already passed through many stages of life with the focus on self-help and learned: We are our own best teachers, healers, and spiritual leaders. Formerly a doctor's assistant, she later studied with a focus on family therapy and gerontology in Frankfurt. She then studied food science in the USA. The dissertation case study on immune defense and Spirulina she published in her bestseller *Spirulina, das blaugrüne Wunder*. The author lived 10 years in the US, intervening in Southern Hesse, Portugal, and Morocco. Until recently, she worked temporarily with maladjusted adolescents in Portugal. She is inspired by a pioneering spirit and a passionate dedication on the well-being of the people.

TABLE OF CONTENT 3

ANALYSIS OF *SPIRULINA PLATENSIS* 7
Preface 8
INTRODUCTION 10

I. WHY DO WE NEED SPIRULINA? 11

Health is a matter of equilibrium 13
Taking Spirulina is especially advisable 15
Preprogrammed vital nutrient deficiency 16
Nutritional deficiency in abundance 16
Food supplements on the increase 17
Spirulina as AIDS prophylaxis in poor countries 18
When do we need more Spirulina? 19
Do we need animal protein? 20
Synthetic is not natural 20
Unique light food for our well-being 22
Spirulina - soul balm for the new era 23
Detox with Spirulina 24

II. FASTING CURE, ENERGIZNG & PERSONALITY FORMNG 26

Spirulina fasting for a basic milieu 26
Colon and liver cleansing: a guarantee for well-being and healing 27
Mitochondrial energy medicine 28
Into a new era of love and light 28

III. *SPIRULINA PLATENSIS* 30

What is Spirulina? 30
Scientific classification of the alga 30
History of the oldest foodstuff 31
Visions and necessity 32
Spirulina dreams to come true ASAP 33
Usage diversity of Spirulina in overview 33
Micro algae breeding by chance 34
   Bringing in the harvest 35
   Dehydration procedure 35
   The pressing of the tablets 35
How to take Spirulina 36
What reactions can occur? 36
Proper storage protects nutrients and biophotons 37

IV. COMPONENTS OF SPIRULINA — 38

- Unique active agents of the blue-green micro algae — 38
- Phycocyanin strengthens the immune system and detoxifies the body — 38
- SOD, *the anti-aging Enzyme* — 39
- Additional leprechauns in action — 40
- Spirulina contains active vitamin B12 — 41
- Beta-carotene as cancer prophylaxis — 41
- Chlorophyll detoxifies and cleanses the blood — 42
- Polysaccharides help to regulate the blood sugar level — 42
- Gamma-linolenic acid inhibits inflammations and regulates hormones — 42
- Sulfolipids and glycolipids act against cancer and AIDS — 43
- Spirulina's vitamins prevent deficiency diseases — 45
- The alga's alkalizing and harmonizing minerals — 47
- Spirulina's unique profile of amino acids — 48

V. SPIRULINA'S HEALTH-PROMOTING EFFECTS — 48

- Why do we live longer than our ancestors? — 49
- Spirulina strengthens your immune system — 49
- The alga helps with hypertension, obesity, and diabetes — 50
- Spirulina detoxes & protects the nerves — 51
- Prompt help for allergic reactions — 51
- The blue-green light carrier cures AIDS — 52
- Spirulina heals wounds and acts as antibiotic — 55
- The micro-organism acts promptly against anemia — 56
- Arthritis: with the blue-green algae rapidly free of complaints — 56
- The alga protects you from eye diseases — 57
- Spirulina prevents acidosis and hair loss — 58
  - *Symptoms of body acidity* — 58
- Spirulina helps to lower cholesterol — 58
- The cyanobacteria has an antidepressant-like effect — 59
- Spirulina stops cancer growth after 3 days — 59
- The miracle alga helps with gastritis and inflammation of the colon — 61
- The *Green Gold* protects the liver and kidneys — 62
- Spirulina protects from radiation damage — 63
- Can components of Spirulina help against tinnitus? — 64

VI. WHO BENEFITS ESPECIALLY FROM SPIRULINA? — 65

- Expectant mothers set the course for their kids' welfare — 65
- Menstruating women often suffer from iron deficiency — 66
- Spirulina: Ritalin ersatz free from side effects — 66
- Vegetarians trust Spirulina as a high quality source of protein — 66
- Permitted doping: power food for heavy workers and athletes — 66
- The elderly living in the fast lane again — 67
- Vital animals with Spirulina as a feed supplement — 68

VII. NATURAL BEAUTY WITH SPIRULINA — 69

Recipes for self-made algae cosmetic — 69
- *Refreshing and lifting poultice* — 69
- *Anti-wrinkle plaster* — 69

Skin and hair poultice — 69
- *Tinted Moisturizer for normal skin* — 69
- *Anti-wrinkle coconut creme* — 70
- *Cream for a firm, full bosom* — 70

Slender and trim with the microalga — 70
Spirulina helps with Cellulite — 70
- *Firming gel* — 70

VIII. SPIRULINA EXPERIENCES AROUND THE GLOBE — 71

Result reports from Germany — 71
Success stories from other countries — 73

IV. RESULTS OF THE ONGOING SPIRULINA STUDY — 75

Improvements by taking Spirulina — 76
The alga in combination with strong drugs — 77
Spirulina related to nutrition and lifestyle — 77

IX. HOW TO USE SPIRULINA IN THE KITCHEN — 79

Recipes — 79

Flavorful meals — 79

- *Bean veggie burger* — 79
- *Chicory salad* — 79
- *Pea puree* — 80
- *Scallion salad* — 80
- *Stewed with vegetable rice* — 80
- *Ginger sesame spread* — 80
- *Chickpeas with "peanut" dressing* — 80
- *Chickpea pie with avocado sauce* — 81
- *Coriander ground patties (vegan)* — 81
- *Lentils pasta with mushroom sauce* — 81
- *Spicy porridge* — 81
- *Red lentil spread* — 82
- *Pesto for the respiratory system* — 82
- *Leftover pancakes* — 82

Sweets without remorse — 82

- *Pineapple kiwi cream* — 82
- *Apricot bars* — 82

Banana cashew cake	83
Figs and sesame patties	83
Lentils granola (gluten-free)	83
Nougat balls	83
Sesame pumpkin pie	83
Sweet carrot casserole	84
Walnut balls	84
Walnut plum bar	84
Citrus almond cake	84

Healthy drinks: turbo power for body, mind and soul	**85**
Drinks for detoxifying your body	85
Coriander and cucumber juice	85
Wild herbs shake	85
Anti-aging goodies to lose weight	86
Kiwi coconut mush	86

Anti-inflammatory drinks	**86**
Fig baobab smoothie	86
Cherries papaya Smoothie	86
Spinach and apple smoothie	86

Liquid soul comforter	**87**
Banana apple shake	87
B vitamin shake	87
Chocolate smoothie	87

Drinks for guts and guns	**87**
Avocado papaya drink	87
Cucumber shake	87
Blueberry smoothie	87
Red currant sorbet	87

Conclusion	**88**
Acknowledgments	**90**
Bibliography	**91**
Index	**95**
QUESTIONNAIRE	**98**

ANALYSIS OF SPIRULINA PLATENSIS

General Data   Average %

Protein	60,8%
Carbohydrates	16,7%
Fat (lipids)	5,3%
Minerals (Ashes)	8,3%
Fibers	6,5%
Moisture	5%

Essential amino acids (g/kg)

Isoleucine	33,8
Leucine	50,1
Lysine	27,5
Methionine	13,7
Phenylalanine	27
Threonine	30
Tryptophane	8,8
Valine	38,7

Non-essential amino acids (g/kg)

Alanine	46,7
Arginine	45
Aspartaic acid	66,9
Cystine	58
Glutamic acid	87,7
Glycine	31,9
Histidine	12,5
Proline	25,9
Serine	29
Thyrosine	26,9

Essential fatty acids (mg/kg)

Linoleic acid	10450
Gamma-Linolenic acid	10633

Pigments and Enzymes (mg/kg)

Carotenoids (orange)	4145
Phycocyanin (blau)	132500
Chlorophyll (grün)	10200
Superoxide dismutase (SOD)	278
Glutathione peroxidase	3,32/g

Nucleic acids (mg/kg)

Ribonucleic acid (RNA)	2,8
Desoxyribonucleic acid (DNS)	0,8

Minerals   (mg/kg)

Magnesium (Mg)	4700
Potassium (K)	4383
Iron (Fe)	10243
Phosphorus (P)	807
Sodium (Na)	8400
Zinc (Zn)	6540
Calcium (Ca)	33
Copper (Cu)	12
Manganese (Mn)	40
Chromium (Cr)	25
Selenium (Se)	1,3
Germanium (Ge)	6
Lithium (Li)	0,35
Molybdenum (Mo)	1,50

Vitamine (mg/kg)

Beta carotene (Provit. A)	1900
Vitamin E (ą-tocopherol)	15
Vitamin B1 (thiamin)	40
Vitamin B2 (riboflavin)	38
Vitamin B3 (niacin)	155
Vitamin B5 (pantothenic acid)	8,3
Vitamin B6 (pyridoxine)	6
Vitamin B12 (cobalamin)	0,4
Folic acid	0,4
Biotin	0,43
Inositol	556,7

Heavy metals (mg/kg)

Arsenic (As)	< 0,10
Lead (Pb)	< 0,29
Cadmium (Cd)	< 0.18
Mercury (Hg)	< 0,01

Herbicides/Pesticides
Not traceable

Microbiology

Gesamtkeimzahl	< 1000KbE/g
Fungi	< 100 KbE/g
Yeast	< 100 kBE/g
Salmonella	nicht nachweisbar (nn)
Staphylococcus	nn
Coliforms	nn

Preface

As a constantly sick child and stuffed with antibiotics I had cataract surgery in both eyes at the age of 13 years. If at the time I would have known that structured water and Spirulina can prevent and cure diseases it would have spared me much suffering. However, it would also have been no motivation to write this book. For, most authors of health books want to help their fellow man not to repeat the own mistakes, but lead a healthy life.

If you trust your inner healer and lead a natural life, you can prevent all suffering and give the doctors and hospitals a wide berth. However, many patients may want to have a greater benefit with rising health insurance costs. Therefore, it would be sensible if we get refunds for not using medical assistance. For this, we could buy Spirulina tablets and psyllium husks powder. With the latter, we can make colon and liver cleansings as shown on page 27 et seq. Because, if the intestine as the important organ of the immune system with 80 % of all immune cells works well, we can enjoy wellness. And, if you take 6 to 8 Spirulina tablets or a tasty beverage from the recipe part during the day, what else should stand in the way of your radiant health? However, if you or a family member are working in the nuclear or chemical industry or in another related risks job you better triple the Spirulina doses.

Taking the immune system boosting microalga and time-shifted psyllium, nature's best fiber, helps you to stay happy, healthy and slim without a scalpel, chemistry, and negative side effects.

If you eat naturally, have enough exercise, fresh air, water, rest and reflection and if you treat yourself with an appropriate activity, you radiate harmony and peace of mind.

Turning your hobby into a profession would be ideal. A Universal Basic Income (UBI) could fulfill this heart's desire of many people. The German dm drugstore boss Götz Werner, for whom the well-being of the employees is more important than the company's return is a supporter of the unconditional basic income. It would also curb the migration of peoples if globally citizens would receive a basic income depending on the economic situation of each country and would be worth the money because it'd get there where it is needed and not spend for favoritism or end up in the pockets of corrupt or lavish statesmen. The German CDU politician Dieter Althaus thinks the unconditional basic income is financially achievable. Applications can be made by Germans online at the following link, and I advise you to ask your elected representative about it.

www.bundesagentur-fuer-einkommen.de

Under the application form you can read this justification for the citizen's income:

*"Technical progress and rationalization are increasingly replacing human labor.
The basic income allows people to participate free, self-responsible and in dignity in this social change process."*

A basic income banks on self-responsibility. With it, you are not authoritative dictated how to behave to be supported by the social policy. It is wiser to give people money so they can decide for themselves instead of doing what they do not want. With a basic income, you can make a career out of your hobby, or you can do more voluntary work. When you enjoy work, you are happy and healthy. We better return to the subject we badly need to stay healthy and healthy. We all need natural food supplements! Because of depleted soils, we are increasingly suffering from nutrient deficiencies.

About 3.6 billion years ago, Spirulina's precursors began to turn the earth into a life-friendly system via photosynthesis. Thus, blue-green algae or cyanobacteria respectively are the mother substance of flora and fauna. Actually, the helical microorganism is not an alga as referred to in the literature. I also use the term algae or microalgae often for the sake of simplicity.

Spirulina contains life-sustaining light particles and countless vital substances, of which probably many have not been discovered yet. Whether as powder or tablets the cyanobacteria help to eliminate pesticides and other pollutants from the body and provide for an enormous vitamin boost. When we eat little meat, we can benefit from Spirulina's high protein content (around 60 %). But before we begin to take the Green Gold it would be advisable to restore the intestine otherwise, the most valuable substances are excreted since they do not even reach the crusty gut walls. Ways and means to clean the intestines and invigorate the body see part II.

During a psychic development seminar in California, I got introduced to Spirulina as a protein food for vegetarians. But only when I was involved in Louise Hay's AIDS-support group and giving Reiki, I realized: Spirulina is more than a dietary supplement. Many of the 300 young men who every Wednesday met in West Hollywood appreciated the light food to strengthen their immune system.

With this book, I would like to show you an alternative to antibiotics and using the bigger guns. Also, I perform ongoing studies with those who have a weak body's defense system. You can find the questionnaire on page 82, or on my website: www.marianne-e-meyer.com. Are you suffering from immunodeficiency and have taken 10 g Spirulina for 4 to 6 weeks, I'd like to ask you to disclose your experiences and send the questionnaire to the address provided or to DrMarianneEMeyer @ gmail. com. If you complete the questionnaire, you'll receive a book with dedication as a thank you.

The microalgae with the scientific name Spirulina platensis contain everything the body needs. You could live only from Spirulina and water. And how could you live! Without the ballast of indigestible food, which leads to the fullness of a Japanese sumo wrestler. Animal products contain a lot of fat and often ferment more than eight hours in the intestines. Thus, they do more harm than good. Antibiotics are mixed with the feed of slaughter animals so they do not become ill and grow faster. They accumulate in the body and form resistant strains. In the case of illness, they are ineffective. A bean burger with Spirulina (page 86) is the healthy alternative to a Big Mac, especially as the filament organism contains three times more protein than meat. Unlike the animal protein, Spirulina's protein is fully digested in about an hour.

Whether you use Spirulina in the kitchen or swallow the pills is up to you. However, I would be pleased if you soon feel better than ever. With Spirulina I have my allergies under control. Colds or cases of flu catch me only very rarely.

The people around me talk about their energy boost, regulated defecation, lower blood sugar, blood pressure, and cholesterol levels, less appetite for sweets. They have rarely pain or anxiety and are balanced with high spirits. They look hopeful into the future and can finally sleep through the night. Cold sores, calluses, acne, lichen and age spots disappear. The skin is moist, soft, and elastic. They have fewer worries about their weight and were physically and mentally never as fit.

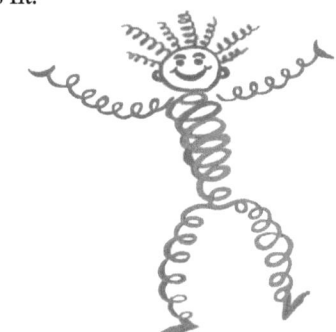

INTRODUCTION

The technical development of the last hundred years, our environment and our way of life changed radically. Not always to the advantage of our planet and all living beings. Every day many plants and animal species die out, and man degenerates rapidly. Therefore, it's about time to set the course or to pull the emergency brake to prevent crueler suffering and more destructive natural disasters. But in this book I make no senseless moral appeals to negligent, oily bilge water bailing captains of rusty oil or chemical tankers that pollute our seas or manufacturers who poison with their waste soil and water. Also, I will sparsely point at the threats of nuclear power plants whose dangerous rest risk could end all our lives. The nuclear disaster at Chernobyl and Fukushima made us terribly aware of this. You will hardly get bored with appeals to human reason to use the bounty of nature to apply environmentally friendly technologies for generating energy. Although these issues are near and dear to me, I concentrate in this compact book on how we can protect ourselves from these and other kinds of dangers with the algae.

As an expert on Spirulina, I want to show you how we all can withstand the stresses of the modern world. With the survival food Spirulina, we can every day anew take the lead. Because the alga is a descendant of the oldest food on earth and therefore it contains all we need. It is capable of eliminating chemical and radioactive substances. It also strengthens the immune system and our inner sewage works.

Our physical and mental environment are overused incessantly by pollutants in the air and the food, addiction, chemical medicines, radio waves, electromagnetic pollution, and stress. Our detox systems run continuously at full speed and can never recover properly. But as we know from experience, if any system can not regenerate, it is eventually prone to interference. In recent years the allergy and cancer rates dramatically increased. This indicates that our body is often pumped up to its neck with poisonous substances. Spirulina platensis, the most researched dietary supplement is an expert to rid the body of toxins. Discover with me what else this miracle of nature can do for your body and mind!

In Part I. you learn how to protect yourself with the detoxifying Spirulina algae from the population-reducing products of the companies Monsanto, Bayer & Co. Further, I explain why nutrient deficiencies are inevitable and when and with which symptoms you need more Spirulina. Also, you can find out why you should prefer the light food over synthetic multivitamins.

In Part II. you learn about the importance of colon and liver cleansing for harmonizing and healing of body, mind, and soul. Because with a crusty gut, the valuable nutrients can hardly reach the blood stream.

Part III provides data on the classification of Spirulina platensis, scientifically known as Arthrospira platensis. But for historical reasons, it is still referred to as Spirulina. Another eye-opener is the history of the oldest food and how native people used it.

Section IV. shows how the vitamins, minerals and unique substances of the alga such as phycocyanin and other pigments, sulfolipids, the anti-aging enzyme SOD and gamma-linolenic acid perform.

Part V. informs how to use the *Green Gold* effectively for your health. It has proven beneficial for allergies, arthritis, eye disease, depression, diabetes, cancer, and much more.

In section VI., you learn who in particular can benefit from Spirulina.

Part VII. is dedicated to homemade Spirulina cosmetics for the skin and hair.

Part VIII. informs you about the amazing experiences of international consumers.

Section IV. shows you the latest results of my ongoing Spirulina study and offers the opportunity to participate in this research by completing the questionnaire.

And last, but not least, you can test your creativity in the recipe part X. by creating delicious meals and drinks. You can use the Spirulina flour every day as a turbo for the body, mind, and soul.

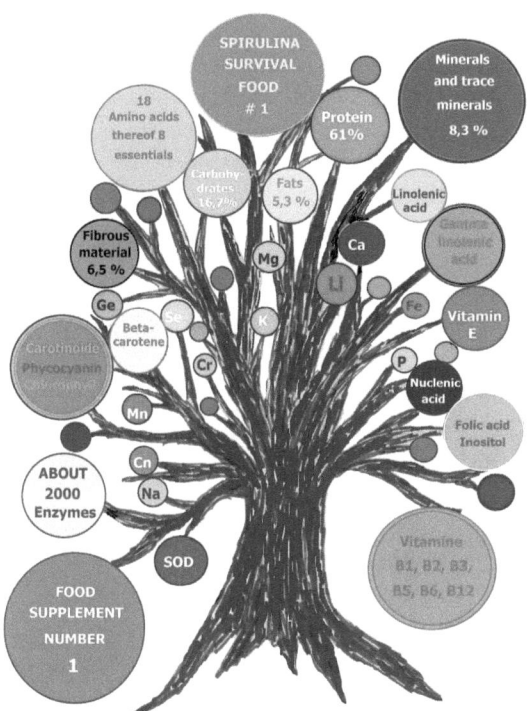

I. WHY DO WE NEED SPIRULINA?

Every day, we breathe in poisons or absorb them through the skin. But most toxins reach the body through our food. Organic food critics argue that it is irrelevant that organic foods contain fewer pesticides than conventional agricultural products, the maximum limits would hardly exceed. However, many pesticides are still insufficiently researched. Let's not allay our alertness. At least for 12 fruits and vegetables, the dirty dozen, Greenpeace is warning, we should resort to organic products. I also recommend to increase the Spirulina ration for detoxification. To cultivate **peppers**, farmers use the chemical ethephon to color them faster. This plant growth regulator acts as a neurotoxin. **Grapes** often contain traces of a poison cocktail with more than 10 different pesticides. Even in **kale**, there is a repeated warning that the limits of pesticides could be exceeded. **Grape leaves** often have critical levels of chemicals. **Cherries** are also often too highly exposed to pesticides. **Pears**, mainly from Turkey, are enormously pesticide-loaded. Growers wash **lettuce** heads in greenhouses and fields with a pesticide shampoo. **Cucumbers** contain a lot of fungicides and insecticides. Conventionally grown **strawberries** bear an abundance of chemicals and pesticides. Crisp, shiny conventionally grown **apples** contain loads of pesticides. Conventional spinach contains enormous amounts of the fertilizer nitrate and listeria.

http://www.greenpeace.org/turkey/Global/turkey/report/2012/04/GPG_Consumer-Guide-Food%20Without%20Pesticides.pdf

You may also reckon that these bacteria are in packaged finished salads. But not only with the diet, we take in toxins, also via cosmetics and especially with the common prescription drugs in traditional medicine. Too many chemical medicines contaminate our body and via wastewater our most important resource, the groundwater.

With the ominous power network of the chemical pharmaceutical industry and medicine today we have no choice but to assume responsibility for our body, our health and thus also for our planet. There is an immensely amount of money to earn with diseases. Thus prevention is not a primary focus in the disease business of western industrialized nations. The ancient Chinese practice of medicine would, however, be ideal: General practitioners were kind of forced to practice preventive medicine. As long as their patients remained healthy, they received a monthly check from them.

After all, the campaign launched by the National Cancer Institute of the USA to daily eat 5 portions of fruit and vegetables reduce the risk of cancer by up to 50% was successful.
http://jn.nutrition.org/content/130/12/3063.full

Other countries followed this recommendation. The British are fighting with heavy artillery and the traffic light colors of red, amber and green on food labels. In Germany, the industry representatives vehemently prevent the traffic light solution for a quick orientation. Politicians in general act against the people's will. On the island, in contrast, since 1.1.2008 are stricter rules on advertising unhealthy foods to children and adolescents in force. The British Heart Foundation (BHF) will reach children with the Food 4 Thought campaign via the Internet, to demonstrate what effect Junk food has on the body and performance:
www.bhf.org.uk/get-involved/campaigning/food4thought.aspx

Often the relationship between diet and disease is negated. For instance, experts continue to discuss the thousands of new breast cancer cases, without ever the word prevention passing their lips. Nutritionists are significantly not invited to these discussions. It would be so easy to prevent breast cancer and other terrible diseases of our questionable civilization with pure water, fresh food, and Spirulina.

If we would compare the diets of nations in relation to their emerging diseases, we could learn a lot in terms of prevention. To stay with breast cancer: In countries with a high milk and meat consumption, women have a higher risk of developing breast cancer. Japanese women who eat traditionally no dairy, little meat, a lot of rice, vegetables, seaweed and fruit, hardly ever get breast cancer. But every year, for about 60 years, near June 1, the world's population is bombarded from the dairy lobby with the same lies. *Milk does a body good!* I remember, when we lived in the US, the dairy industry had to change their formerly slogan milk does *the* body good in does *a* body good. It is especially alarming that in the equally old diet rules called Codex Alimentarius, an outgrowth of world domination, the war criminal Fritz ter Meer was involved. He was responsible for the Auschwitz-industrial site of IG Farben, and after the prison term, he returned to the Supervisory Board of Bayer AG, the company that is buying Monsanto! Dr. Mathias Rath counts the Codex Alimentarius to the grossest violations of human rights in history.
www4.dr-rath-foundation.org/PHARMACEUTICAL_BUSINESS/health_movement_against_codex/health_movement24.htm

Can you imagine: This food book was architected by the chemical and pharmaceutical industry and a war criminal, and all countries are committed to it through a trade agreement. This also includes food labeling regulations. E. g., if a country would decide against GM corn or its labeling, it would face an immensely high penalty. There seems to be no true democracy on this planet. The people's will is no GM corn nor its regulation by not labeling. Who wants something on the plate which is known to create tumors and liver and kidney damage? In 2012 Gilles-Eric Séralini and his French colleagues have fed rats for two years with the also in Europe approved corn variety NK 603 from Monsanto and control. They discovered the rodents receiving the GM corn had increased liver and kidney damage. Similarly, these animals developed more tumors and died earlier than the control group.

http://www.gmoseralini.org/wp-content/uploads/2012/11/GES-final-study-19.9.121.pdf

Better red than dead? Immediately after learning of the study, Russia banned the import of genetically modified corn. In the rest of the world, the study is controversial. GM corn recommending lobbyists accused the researchers but without success. What else are we to expect from the designers of the new world order? Readers of my age may have noticed that half a century ago the problem of overpopulation was ever discussed while today we hear little about it. Is the solution to the problem already in the works? Is the goal of the global elite our physical and mental poisoning and enslavement? Do we have to protect ourselves from Rockefeller, Gates & Co? If so, how is this to be achieved? We better question everything unnatural, and closely check certain studies and the response to them. Such as the one of Arpad Pusztai, who investigated GM potatoes on behalf of the Scottish Agriculture Environment and Fisheries Department. The rats his team fed with GM potatoes had significantly smaller organs including the testicles and brains as well as a weak immune system. Blair and Clinton should have called personally to prevent the publication of the study. Why Pusztai was fired along with his team and their results should have been suppressed is left to the reader.

http://www.psrast.org/pusztblair.htm

In 2005, the Vereinigung Deutscher Wissenschaftler (Federation of German Scientists) awarded him the Whistleblower price.

How do we protect us against such malicious power structures? In everything, we are presented with we better listen to our inner voice and ask who benefits from it? Cui bono? Let's not take us for a fool! And we better think seriously about hoarding seeds and protect us with organic fruits, vegetables, and Spirulina, the power food in its purest form. The microorganism needs little acreage and resources. Jean-Paul Jourdan shows you how you can grow the blue-green microalgae.

www.antenna.ch/en/documents/Jourdan_UK.pdf

You need for the production in addition to the cultures a food-safe plastic wrap, a few solar panels and a starter from a scrap car. With this and a lot of sunshine you can make environmentally friendly and energy saving the best food in the world. Even near my university city Frankfurt people grow Spirulina.

Since the algae remove toxins, heavy metals, and even radioactive substances from the body, you have some protection with daily consumption. The health condition of Japanese seems to prove this statement. They consume 10-15 % and have the longest life expectancy in spite of the nuclear bombs dropped on Japan in 1945. But when researching for the Cranberry book, I noticed that most of the Methuselah, people who are more than 100 years old, live in countries where people drink traditionally cranberry juice and eat cranberries.

Health is a matter of equilibrium

Due to denatured foods and increasing environmental pollution, the body needs to fight off increasingly aggressive free radicals. These unstable molecules in the most aggressive manner snatch away electrons from fats, carbohydrates, proteins, nucleic acids, and even from genetic substance coding nucleic acids. To regain balance the robbed molecules now attack other compounds leading to a chain reaction. If free radicals can no longer be repelled by the body's protective system, oxidation stress originates, causing imbalance and illness.

Despite a scavenger protection system, healthy nutrition, and a healthy lifestyle, we can hardly neutralize all free radicals nowadays. Therefore, it is strongly advisable to compensate for the increased need for antioxidants with food supplements. Spirulina contains only small amounts of the most potent antioxidant superoxide dismutase (SOD) but the minerals zinc, copper, and manganese which the body needs for the production of this enzyme. It also contains other biocatalysts and beta-carotene, vitamin E, selenium and a number of other free-radical scavengers. If we assume the creation makes no mistakes we can presuppose:

Diseases, even those caused by injuries, are usually based on material or spiritual poisoning.

All the symptoms are an effort of the organism to get rid of toxins and to bring the body chemistry back into balance. As nature strives for balance and harmony, we need to do nothing else than to assist our body in the elimination of toxic substances. Sick animals drink plenty of water and eat grass. We also need to detoxify with water. Everything the grass contains and much more, you can obtain from the blue-green micro-algae Spirulina. But if efforts to excrete the toxins through the intestines, urinary tract, respiratory tract and skin are suppressed with chemical drugs, even more pollutants accumulate in the body. The immune system may be so overwhelmed that the white blood cells are busy with the neutralization of the toxins. It can not handle germs and cancer cells we constantly pick up. Or the congested body defense goes crazy, and the white blood cells attack instead of toxic debris endogenous proteins and cause autoimmune/autoaggressive diseases. These include Hashimoto, MS, and rheumatism.

As is known algae excrete heavy metals and other toxins. Carotene-containing vegetables reduce the risk of getting cancer.

In today's rush more and more people resort to fast food. But to prevent disease, it would be advisable to daily peel carrots, clean broccoli, cook vegetable soups and make salads. But today who takes time for the traditional preparation of meals? Despite the cooking show's boom, the temptations of the countless convenience foods are ample. We could consume a prepared dish every single day of the year. But we need no intensified gray cells acrobatics to realize that this repeatedly heated devitalized and with artificial substances preserved stodge does our body more harm than good. At least, with the preservatives, we remain alive longer, because not only the food is preserved, also everybody who consumes it. Only it is rather a painful frailty associated with the loss of feet or legs in diabetes, aching rheumatism and other degenerative conditions. If we eat raw vegetables and fruits, we relieve the pancreas with the including food enzymes: You must then produce fewer enzymes ergo biocatalysts. Without fresh food, it bleeds dry, and the glucose level in the blood rises.

What can we do to link the demands of our time with our body's need for valuable nutrients? We could research ourselves with the wonder algae. Who should have a greater interest than ourselves? In the health-oriented public, natural food supplements are considered the silver lining on the horizon. And the positive effects on the organism are in no way based on placebo effects.

Animals also benefit from Spirulina (see chapter: Vital animals with Spirulina as a feed supplement.

The detoxifying, cancer preventive and cancer-inhibiting algae contain many vital substances in a concentrated form. E. g., the defense strengthening pigments phycocyanin, carotenoids, and chlorophyll, the rare, in breast milk occurring anti-inflammatory gamma-linolenic acid and the aforementioned anti-aging enzyme SOD.

- Japanese women rarely consume milk and hardly suffer from breast cancer.

- Illnesses are in general due to material and spiritual poisoning of the body and soul. Symptoms are efforts of the organism to rid itself of toxins.

- Gourmands need Spirulina for discharging pollutants. Who receives little fresh vegetables, salad, and fruit needs the alga for the prevention of cancer, diabetes, and other mass epidemics.

- Canned pre-cooked dishes are no life-sustaining foods.

- Spirulina contains except vitamin C all vital substances plus unique, immune potentiating, anti-cancer and anti-inflammatory antioxidants: phycocyanin, SOD, gamma-linolenic acid, carotenoids and much more.

Taking Spirulina is especially advisable
- when you eat little green and yellow fruit and vegetables
- if you use sugar, cigarettes or alcohol
- if you lack energy and motivation
- when your moods fluctuate
- with problems getting to sleep
- if you suffer from dizziness (anemia or low blood sugar)
- with frequently occurring cold sores
- If you have pale, prematurely aged skin and lackluster, brittle hair and nails
- with aphthous ulcers, warts or athlete's foot
- if you are night-blind
- with nervousness, anxiety & hyperactivity
- with allergies and frequent infections
- if you desire certain foods
- if in your family cancer propagates
- in old age, as the immune system of the elderly weakens

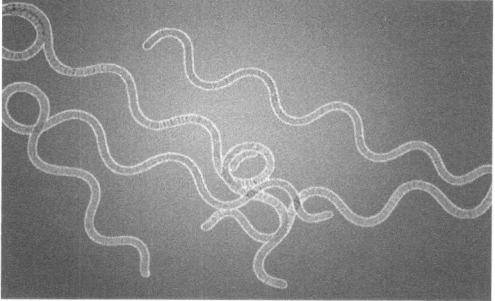

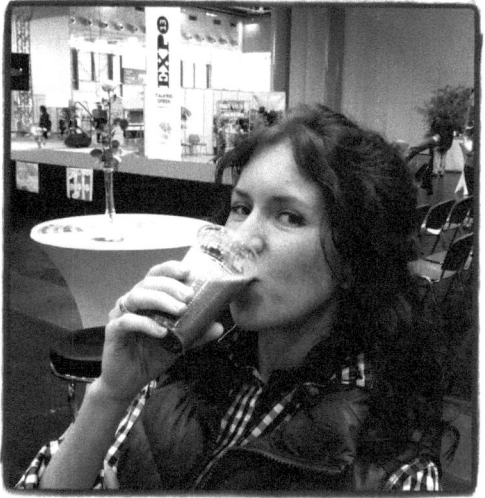

Anissa Brauneis treats herself at the stand of a known Spirulina company to a Spirulina mint smoothie.

http://www.anissabrauneis.at

Pre-programmed vital nutrient deficiency

100 years ago, we were still 90 % involved with our muscle power on the so-called total energy supply. Our ancestors had to work hard for their livelihood: rub the wash, scrub the floor, shake all the rugs, collect wood and chop, haul buckets of water, collect mushrooms and berries. Today, we think of more sophisticated methods to avert physical exertion. Therefore, the rate has slipped below 1%. Physical work often remains just in using the muscles of mastication. Prof. Rozalind Gruben warns: The most important factor leading to porous bones is the lack of exercise. Because, if muscles do not pull on bones, the latter have no reason to remain strong (1999). Also:

Lacking of movement perfuses the brain poorly. Lymph, toxins, and waste products are not eliminated efficiently.

Only if all body fluids are in flux, we are healthy and balanced. This implicates to drink enough structured water. I refine my tap water with an award-winning water activation technology (Meyer 2015). Lack of exercise leads to obesity and nutritional deficits. Junk food, coffee, cigarettes, chemical drugs, illegal drugs, radioactive rays, exhaust fumes and other environmental toxins empty out your vital nutrient storage. Many people eat fatty ready-to-eat meals or warmed-up white-flour dishes in cafeterias and consume many sugars in solid and liquid form. Such foods contain harmful stress vitamin robbers. The lack of vitamin B5 (pantothenic acid) leads to abdominal pain and muscle spasms. When rushing to the doctor and taking chemical drugs, more valuable nutrients are lost.

• Our body needs daily exercise to strengthen the bones, increase the blood flow in the brain and eliminate pollutants.

• Tobacco and environmental toxins rob the body vitamins and salts.

• Chemical drugs attack the last vital nutrient reserves.

Nutritional deficiency in abundance

The nutrition report of the Deutsche Gesellschaft für Ernährung (German Society for Nutrition) informs among other things about the nutritional content of our blood. Accordingly, men and women of almost all ages are missing calcium, magnesium, vitamin E, carotenoids, folic acid and other nutrients. Many menstruating women furthermore suffer from iron deficiency. Even if we eat a balanced diet, we can suffer from lack of nutrients. How come? In the Brockhaus:

Crop rotation thus the succession of different agricultural products to certain principles (cropping) is essential to prevent soil fatigue, pests, and disease.

That may sound reasonable but is bad for business. Therefore, the modern agriculture gave it up. Thus our arable land is exhausted. Ergo our food is lacking selenium and other essential trace elements. Fatal vital nutrient deficiency is the result. Our failure to compensate for these deficiencies with food supplements will result in much higher cancer rates and other diseases. But this is only half the terrifying truth. Namely, when the natural pest is eliminated by lacking crop rotation, conventionally growing farmers fight the pests with pathogenic pesticides. Consequently, we permanently get poisoned.

Parkinson is a disease related to pesticides. Spirulina is proven to eliminate toxins, and their anti-inflammatory potential may also inhibit inflammation in the brain, associated with Parkinson.

Spirulina is useful in three ways: as fertilizer, natural pest control, complemental vital substance concentrate to compensate for nutritional deficiencies and as a detox aid to eliminate pollutants.

As long as we do not get naturally grown crops, the nutritious alga is an excellent alternative to prevent nutritional deficiencies.

- Iron, calcium, magnesium, vitamin E, carotenoids, and folic acid are usually lacking substances in women of childbearing potential.
- The absence of crop rotation causes the soil to lack minerals. Spirulina compensates for the loss of vital substances and eliminates pesticides and other pollutants.
- Pesticides have to do with our modern epidemics such as Parkinson's, Alzheimer's, autism, asthma, reproductive disorders, diabetes, and cancer.

Food supplements on the increase

Like all that is new spills across the big pond, food supplements also reached Europe. Its history goes back some 70 years. In the working-class neighborhoods of Pittsburgh, citizens ate a diet predominantly deprived of B vitamins: polished rice, toast and other white bread. Because of this shortage of nutrients, particularly the B vitamins and trace elements, many Pittsburghers were ill. Some landed in psychiatric care.

Biochemically oriented doctors and health practitioners, who did not treat just the symptoms, achieved astonishing healing successes with supplementing lacking nutrients. Thus, the topic dietary supplement has been driven by the US scientists.

Our fundamental diet change calls for concentrated nutrients. Frozen and canned foods, pizzas, and burgers and what else snack bars or fast food restaurants offer today are our sad reality. The traditional preparation of food with selected natural ingredients fades into the background. While prominent TV chefs on all channels are trying to create an awareness of healthy choices, they mostly must rely on the same crops of depleted soil. This and the modern food production are the cause that we suffer increasingly from nutrient deficiency diseases and depend on superfoods such as Spirulina, cereal grasses, and weeds. Our foods are often no more food but vegetate means. Rarely blessed by the sun, they contain little vitality. And biochemically, the valuable husks of the grains are removed. Artificially processed foods barely supply nutrients to our cells. The worthless fare agglutinates our intestinal walls and lays the foundation for the suffering of our questionable civilization.

In India, every seventh person with psychiatric disorders suffers from a lack of various B vitamins, caused by an unbalanced diet with polished rice. Without sufficient amounts of these nerve-strengthening vitamins, neither the brain functions normally nor the nervous system remains stable. By compensating nutrient deficiencies with natural food supplements like Spirulina, significantly fewer patients would vegetate in psychiatric hospitals. This verified physicians at the US East Coast. In the Princeton Bio Brain Center in New Jersey, they treated 5000 applicable schizophrenic patients on an outpatient basis until the 1990s under the direction of Dr. Carl C. Pfeiffer. 90% could be socially fully rehabilitated through whole foods and dietary supplementation with specific nutrients.

Spirulina contains all the micronutrients used to treat different types of schizophrenia, e. g., niacin (Vitamin B3), pyridoxine (B6), zinc and manganese for mental diseases caused by hypoglycemia (low blood sugar). Almost half of US-Americans use dietary supplements to compensate for nutritional deficiencies, usually inorganic vitamins, and mineral tablets. But the organism has problems assimilating inorganic salts. Over time they accumulate in the filter of the connective tissue, in the joints and arteries. Japanese use organic food supplements such as blue-green algae, kelp, kombu, arame, wakame, nori, dulse and other algae. Therefore, the Japanese are healthier and have in international comparison the highest life expectancy. They live about five years longer than people in other industrialized nations. How come? As already mentioned, Japanese consume traditionally little milk and animal products, such as raw fish in sushi, but the whole range of edible seaweed. We consider these in the water growing plants as exotic delicacy or food supplements. In the Asian cuisine, they are an integral part. Hopefully, the recent nuclear disaster in Japan had also little impact on public health due to this elimination diet. Since the Fukushima fallout burdened the Pacific coast of the United States and other regions, we would be well advised to all consume Spirulina and other edible algae on a regular base.

In addition to malnutrition, we have to deal with much higher stress and increased environmental toxins, since the construction of nuclear plants. Because of the higher radiation doses, detoxifying food supplements such as Spirulina are essential. You can also collect wild herbs in exhaust emissions-free areas. See also chapter *Detox with Spirulina.*

• The history of dietary supplements began in the working class neighborhoods of Pittsburgh: The consumed white rice and toast led to vitamin B deficiency.

• The lack of B- (stress vitamins) leads to mental suffering.

• Spirulina contains all the micronutrients used for the natural treatment of mental illness.

• Japanese women have the highest life-expectancy. Japanese eat 10 to 15% algae. This detoxifying diet protects the body from disease.

Spirulina as AIDS prophylaxis in poor countries

Worldwide we produce twice as many foods as the world population needs. Yet, every year millions of children die from the effects of malnutrition and related immune deficiency. In developing countries, more than 100,000 children go blind every year due to the lack of vitamin A; approximately a quarter is suffering from severe iron deficiency anemia, the main cause of immunodeficiency.

Although the United Nations agency UNICEF, Terre des Hommes and other facilities offer help for children in poor countries, the proportion of underweight children under 5 years was between 1990 and 2010 only reduced by 2.6 %. The mortality rate declined only slightly. 230 million children under 15 years are still suffering from malnutrition and related immunodeficiency. Their foods consisting of rice, corn or millet contain few calories, protein, and nutrients. These deficiencies have irreparable consequences for the children's further development. As adults, they are weak and suffer physical and or mental disabilities.

How can children receive their right to the highest attainable standard of health in accordance with the article 24 of the UN convention? The key to human fulfillment lies in its autonomy. Regardless of material resources, man can gather information and develop. Give a man a fish, and you feed him for a day; show him how to catch fish, and you feed him for a lifetime. The non-governmental organization Antenna Technology found a way to escape from the vicious circle with the nutrient-rich algae: because the daily addition of only 1 g Spirulina is sufficient to stimulate metabolic processes and promote growth.

This, among other things, was demonstrated by researchers at the Children's Hospital of Madurai in South India with 60 malnourished children. Therefore, Antenna decided to induce the cultivation of blue-green algae in the area. It arose a pilot project of Spirulina growing securing the food needs of more than a thousand children and at the same time representing an income opportunity. Furthermore, women get the opportunity to learn the basics in a healthy diet. There were also low effort growing programs developed where they are most needed. To enable as many regions and countries in the developing world to benefit from their actions, Antenna is dependent on financial aid. More and more villages want to grow Spirulina as they can prevent malnutrition only at a local level. The children get stirred in a ration of Spirulina powder into their daily pulp supplying them with the necessary nutrients. Here, you can get involved:

www.antenna.ch/en

African doctors prescribe their AIDS patients the immune-boosting algae because they found out that the T-helper lymphocytes (CD4 lymphocytes) increased in people who had taken Spirulina.

During HIV infection, CD4 (positive) lymphocyte decline continuously. The CD4 count (CD = cluster of differentiation) is thus an important prognostic parameter for the acquired immune deficiency. African doctors recognized that Spirulina increases the CD4 helper cells and thus boosts the immune system. Based on the information on the internet and in my books, fewer people obtain prescriptions for cell killing chemical drugs that bring the body out of balance and lead to fatal side effects. This is why the immune deficiency is spreading less than expected.

http://www.antenna.ch/en/research/nutrition

Our visions of integral life and coexistence can flourish even in the planned international southern Indian city of Auroville. There are currently living 2,184 people from 50 nations. The citizens of the future city also cultivate Spirulina, the food of the future.

www.auroville.org/health/food/spirulina.htm

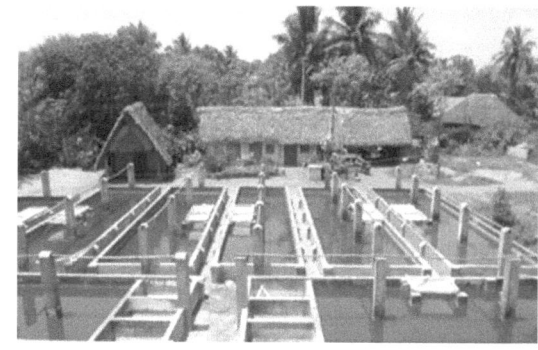

- Annually, 6 million infants die from malnutrition and disease.
- Antenna technology developed Spirulina cultivation programs to secure a vital substance food supply at the local level.
- African doctors found that Spirulina increases the CD4 helper cells and thus strengthens the immune system.

When do we need more Spirulina?

At certain times it is advisable to increase the dose of 3 to 5 g Spirulina, namely:

- Before physical and mental exertion
- In times of increased risk of disease:
- During cold periods and hormonal changes: during puberty, pregnancy, and menopause
- Before or after radiation treatments or X-ray examinations or during chemotherapy, since the alga protects against radiation and eases side effects
- Before or after intercontinental flights to protect against radiation exposure in the highlands or in countries blessed with the sunshine as UV-radiation protection
- Before the menses, against premenstrual suffering and as iron deficiency prophylaxis
- Between meals for blood sugar balance
- On longer trips by car if there is traffic congestion, to prevent heavy metal poisoning

- With heavy alcohol or tobacco consume to support the detox organs and to balance vital substance losses
- With strains, that curb the immune system such as shock situations, times of sadness, fear of examinations or constant stress
- During convalescence after severe suffering or accidents
- To support traditional, ungentle treatment methods: to avoid side effects and blood poisoning
- Before and after each visit to the dental doctor when he works with amalgam or other toxins or give injections

Do we need animal protein?

Many people eat sausage and meat because they believe that a diet without animal protein is harmful. The situation is rather the opposite: The consumption of meat, sausage, and cheese in the quantities consumed today endangers our health! Also, our body can not cope with the cattle's feed additions: Dioxin, PCB chlorine, antibiotics, growth hormones and many more problematic substances found during inspections. The scandals do not stop. Countless animals have already fallen victim to them. We can assume that people who consume large quantities of animal products without eating greens and drinking pure water, the detoxification organs become seriously ill. This shows how much we need the detox alga Spirulina. Studies show: Vegetarians are more powerful and have more endurance than meat eaters. A surprising number of top athletes are vegetarians, like Patrick Baboumian, the strongest man (2011), the Ex-tennis stars Boris Becker and Martina Navratilova as well as the legendary country distance runner Paavo Nurmi who earned nine gold medals. Also, most spiritual leaders eat predominantly meatless.

Leonardo da Vinci, Nikola Tesla, Mahatma Gandhi and Albert Einstein were vegetarians.

Anyone who is uncertain or believes, legumes, seeds nuts, and weeds do not produce sufficient protein, rely safely on the alga: Spirulina is the best protein source the planet has to offer. Since its fossil predecessor once planted the greenhouse soil, the cyanobacteria are on the cusp between plants and animals. As plant related bacterium it is close to the animal and therefore contains enough cobalamin (vitamin B12), to meet the minimum daily requirement of three micrograms. But we better not take Spirulina with other B12-containing foods. Because it supposedly contains about two-thirds B12 analogs, pseudo-vitamin B12. Those can block the absorption of vitamin B12. See also chapter Spirulina contains active vitamin B12.

• Vegans consume only vegetable protein and are considered healthy and productive.

• Athletes such as Carl Lewis, Edwin Moses, and Torre Washington eat pure organic.

• Plants often do not contain complete protein and have to be combined: rice and beans or cereal with nuts.

• Spirulina's protein is the most valuable and most becoming ever; the digestive time is less than an hour.

• The cyanobacterium contains enough vitamin B12 to meet the minimum daily requirement of 3 micrograms. See page 41.

Synthetic is not natural

From the ancient times on, people have trusted in the healing effects of nature. Diseases, which are known to be primarily caused by the body's poisoning, healed with fasting and herbs until some brain acrobats had the profane idea artificial remedies would have to be better than natural ones. In the course of time, the more complex the construction of chemical compounds, the more valuable it could be resulting in a flourishing pharmaceutical industry. Many

Protein Parts Compared	
Spirulina	61%
Soybeans	34%
Limburger cheese	30%
Linseed	24%
Legumes	22%
Salami	22%
Nuts	15 - 25%
Fish	17 - 25%
Red meat	15 - 25%
Poultry	18 - 21%
Hen's egg	12%
Quark	11 - 13%
Wheat flour type 405	10%
Rice	7%

Hoffmann (Hrsg.) Positivlisten Lebensmittel

physicians discovered new diseases caused by the side effects of chemical remedies decorating them with their names. Thus, clinical dictionaries grew into a host of imposing symptom complexes. The creators of such miracles, some of which no longer see the forest from the trees, were glorified as white gods.

The medicine turned increasingly against creation. Natural products with a preventive and healing effect were henceforth considered critical. Today we tend to be skeptical when something is simple and natural yet heals. Especially if it is a food promise wonders. Here the founder of scientific medicine Hippocrates said around 2500 years ago, our food should be our medicine. Synthetic food and synthetic food supplements, on the other hand, lead to allergies or death. Dangerous are especially artificial sweeteners and flavor enhancers. Aspartame (E951), also known as AminoSweet, NutraSweet, Equal, and Canderel, can not be metabolized by all people. It sometimes leads to headaches and dizziness. Neurosurgeon Russell L. Blaylock stated:

Aspartame and glutamic acid cause serious chronic neurological disorders and are responsible for countless symptoms and diseases: epilepsy, MS, Parkinson's, Alzheimer's, brain tumor, blindness, carbuncles, depression, impaired short-term memory or reduction of intellectual capacity.

In the US, consumer groups have set up a hotline for Aspartame victims. Stevia is a healthy alternative to artificial sweeteners. Until a few years ago Germans had to buy it as bath additive since it was not approved as food. For many years the Japanese sweeten more than half their foods and drinks with Stevia, also cola. In the US you could buy it as a nutritional supplement until 2008. Meanwhile, Stevia is allowed as a safe sugar substitute. Due to the hitherto longer life expectancy of the Japanese no one apparently wanted to say, Stevia is healthwise questionable.

On the other hand, it is clung tightly to Aspartame, although several studies have revealed the artificial sweetener as a carcinogen entailing a higher risk of premature birth. So why is Aspartame considered safe? Fortunately, we can still decide for ourselves as consumers!

In the fall of 2010, German TV viewers were informed by TV chef Tim Mälzer that almost all spice mixes, salad dressings, and soups include monosodium glutamate (E 621, also declared as flavor, aroma or yeast extract). So if you suffer from restless legs and restless sleep, you better read the fine print on the packages carefully. The suffering caused by the artificial foods is piling up! So some contemporaries carry bad karma which they have burden themselves with through the creation of suffering. The problem with Aspartame is known for decades. On 04/11/2004 suits were filed against several companies that manufacture or use Aspartame in their products on three courts in California. More info at: prweb.com/releases/2004/4/prweb117841.php

Artificial food coloring and preservatives acidify our body fluids and if the elimination channels are congested, accumulate in the tissues and joints. If you want to get or stay healthy, there is only one way: back to nature! From cyanobacteria, flora and fauna developed including any herbal remedy. The overriding importance of health and the numerous healing effects of the beneficial microalgae is not, therefore such a great miracle. Because, as water and cyanobacteria were at the beginning of everything, we can obtain whatever our body lacks from water and Spirulina. At the beginning of the modern era, the development of herbal medicine was interrupted. Chemical preparations have been developed. Due to the side effects of synthetic drugs allergic reactions and other immune deficiency diseases formed.

- The academical world destroyed the people's trust in the natural remedies. The patients transferred the responsibility for their bodies to medical school.
- With the increasing poisoning, doctors are often at their wits' end, and the run in the natural medicine followed.
- From cyanobacteria, the plants and animals developed. Therefore, we can compensate dietary deficiencies with Spirulina.
- Aspartame, E 621-25, and other food chemicals cause a variety of ailments.

Unique light food for our well-being

Already Akhenaten in Ancient Egypt had known about the special healing powers of the sun. The sunlit food, whether animal or plant, gives us energy and vitality. The Swiss Dr. M. Bircher-Benner and later Prof. W. Kollath expressed that sunlight provides the actual nutritional value in food. Artificially irradiated agricultural products are dead means. They may be more durable but do us more harm than good. The more light energy (biophotons) foods can store the higher the quality. The pioneer of biophotons Prof. Fritz A. Popp suggests that the ability to store biophotons must be a measure of the quality of our food (1988, 1993). Naturally grown vegetables and sun-ripened fruits have extensively refueled solar energy. Monika Helmke Hausen affirms, fruits touch us in essence, strengthen the soul and let our knowledge shine in us. The latter may also cause the water contained therein.

The microalgae store a lot of light energy. In their thin filaments with blue, green and orange pigments can, contrary to the plants green of the leaves, absorb the entire light spectrum. Biophotons measurements of weak light emissions from biological organisms confirm:

Spirulina is an excellent storage of solar power. The absorbed solar energy is available for the body in the form of biophotons. These tiny light particles pass through the food in our cells. They contain important bio information controlling complex life processes in our body. Not the calories' energy is crucial but the info.

Popp considers food as a remedy, transferring the missing vibrations to the organism. So, it is only logical to conclude: The ultra-weak light is supporting the exchange of information between the cells or the intracellular water. The so-called light water, e. g., the Lourdes water from the Pyrenees or the water of the Hunzas from the Himalayas have unusual frequencies working positively on the organism. Spirulina also contains the entire light spectrum from blue-violet to red. These biophotons have an organizing and regulating effect bringing the body to a higher vibration and order which is expressed by vitality and well-being. Think about greenhouses, battery hens, and animals for fattening! No solar energy is coming into the food thus doing us more harm than good.

In a blind test of the Landesuntersuchungsanstalt in Celle, Barbara Köhler presented significant differences in the light storage capability of free range eggs to eggs from battery cages.*) With the same feed, the eggs showed biochemically no difference. Therefore we can assume that the overall state of the biophotons and not the chemical reaction of the components determines the quality of food (Popp, 1988, Köhler et al. 1991).

Food that does not store sunlight is of little use for the human organism. This is, why today many people hang around tired, don't know what to do and messing around.

Yet it may not be desirable to replace meals with Spirulina dishes. But you can enjoy the light food par excellence as a snack in the form of a delicious banana-apple shake or a delicious fruit bar. Even if we flush down the stimulating tablets with a glass of water, we affect the desire for green stuff. Thus, we do something good for us and our animal friends, who we need to torment less.

• Spirulina provides the organism with useful light frequencies.

• Free range eggs deliver solar power; eggs from battery cages harm the body.

• The protein-containing light food curbs the appetite for animal products.

*)Since 2012 it is prohibited in the EU to keep laying hens in traditional cage systems. In Germany, since 2010 no more poultry is kept in cages. Take care the USA and the UK will ban it too.

Spirulina - soul balm for the new era

In addition to the daily news, tablets for high blood pressure, heartburn (antacids), pain, water pills and some heart medication and antibiotics can make indirect depressed.

Spirulina helps to lift the spirits. The algae tablets remind of the cheering up pills that make the life easier in Aldous Huxley's Brave New World. In a doomsday mood, we are asked by the English-speaking, do you have the blues. The blues originate predominantly from the weather conditions. Lack of sun rays, foehn, but also stomach overflow, poor diet and lack of exercise can also cause the blues. They can develop into depression and melancholy. Should the bogeymen pounce on you and the pendulum swings between gnawing pain and choking fear, it's time for Spirulina. South Korean scientists warn us to take the algae. Because they are exploring at the University of Seoul, the antidepressant effect of Spirulina in a forced swimming test with mice. Their results suggest that it acts as antidepressants (Kim 2008).

Because it contains the cheering up and antidepressant amino acids phenylalanine, tyrosine, and tryptophan. Also, their B vitamins have a positive effect on our nerves. Niacin (B3) improves the blood circulation and helps fight depression and schizophrenia. The antistress vitamin pantothenic acid (B5) helps, especially against anxiety and depression. Pyridoxine (B6) supports the nervous system. The cobalamin (B12) and the glycolipids in Spirulina build the protective layer of the nerve cells or the myelin sheaths respectively. The minerals calcium and magnesium help against depression. They provide for the reduction of stress acids and for strong nerves. So it is no wonder that Spirulina helps immediately to a mood uplift. It also helps with eczema, afflicting today many children. Mechanical or environmental influences can cause endogenous or atopic eczema. But too much hygiene, allergies or a fermenting gut are rarely the sole cause. In 1998, Buser and his research colleagues from Hannover Medical School found out in a study with 4219 preschoolers that in the expensive residential areas up to a quarter of the children suffer from itchy eczema. In the poorer neighborhoods, there are only about 3%. Sterility and achievement orientation with stressful thoughts, not to make it can create disharmony. In children with a migrant background, the pressure to perform appears to be less because they suffer less from neurodermatitis. The alkaline minerals, B vitamins, and other components in Spirulina sooth stress and provide for good nerves, emotional balance, and a strong self-confidence.

- The moral booster Spirulina leads to joy and harmony.
- The high vitamin B content and the alkaline minerals help with stress and prevent eczema, depression, and schizophrenia.
- The cobalamin (vitamin B_{12}) and the glycolipids protect the nerves.

Detox with Spirulina

For half a century the stresses from environmental toxins in the overcrowded industrial areas have leaped. Lead is one of the most dangerous environmental toxins. It enters the body through air, food, and water. Who gets too little calcium, iron, and protein with the food, is in danger of absorbing too much lead or cobalt through the gastrointestinal tract. The heavy metals enter the blood, circulating bound to amino acids and accumulate mainly in the bone tissue, liver, and kidney.

Spirulina contains in well-measured, high quality and bioavailable form exactly those substances which promote the elimination of lead and strengthen the immune system: healing frequencies of light, 60% high-grade, easily digestible protein, calcium, magnesium, iron, selenium, sulfur-containing amino acids and the vitamins A, B, and E. These nutrients as well as SOD and other enzymes reduce the toxic effect of free radicals and protect our cells from oxidizing.

In Belarus, 16 workers loaded with lead received 5 Spirulina tablets per day as a dietary supplement. For all women, the lead levels in the blood and urine decreased. After two months, the MAD-level was significantly lower and showed normal WHO values.

A negative consequence of lipid peroxidation is the formation of Malondialdehyde (MAD). This aldehyde binds with protein and forms insoluble complexes that accumulate in the cells and this can cause damage.

It showed increasing important enzymes in the lipid oxidation system and antioxidant system. The lead line to the teeth disappeared. The tissue condition of the gums and enhanced susceptibility to infection in the oral cavity decreased. With this, the researchers Loseva and Urinok of the clinic of the Research Institute of Radiation Medicine and Endocrinology in Minsk proved that the consumption of Spirulina as a food supplement acts exuding with lead poisoning.

Many international scientists were able to prove the heavy metal absorbing effect of the alga. Researchers from the Department of Chemistry at the Iowa State University were able to verify Spirulina's enormous absorbing biological and physicochemical activity against mercury ions (Cain et al. 2007). Therefore, many dentists, holistic doctors, and health practitioners use the algae in elimination. The study also indicates the benefit of Spirulina as a daily dietary supplement in industrialized countries with regard to disease prevention. (Naturheilpraxis 5/2000). In further studies with Chernobyl children was found that the alga is even able to excrete radioactive rays. Thus it can reduce the fear of people of radioactive radiation. See part *Spirulina protects from radiation damage.*

Drug or alcohol abuse and toxins in food or the environment can lead to inflammation of the liver. Spirulina has a regenerative effect on the detox organs. It helps to reduce the negative side effects of drug treatments since it purifies the blood and relieves the elimination organs. If you daily use drinks and tobacco you need the healing and regenerating algae regularly. Also, if you daily consume coffee, chocolate and ice cream. Even the excessive consumption of sugar with milk can lead to a fatty liver and poor liver function. Mixing milk and sugar leads to fermentation and produces fusel alcohols in the body, resulting in acidosis and weak liver and kidneys. In addition to the excretory function, Spirulina reduces the addictive behavior, especially cravings for sweets. Since sugar is a vitamin B and calcium robber, Spirulina also protects nerves and bones.

It would also be wise to consume the algae before or after each x-ray treatment for the withdrawal and prevention of suffering. Diabetes, blood disorders, cardiovascular disease, stroke, and cataracts are related to x-rays. Also, the side effects of drugs can have frightening consequences. Our body should serve us as long as possible. Therefore we better are careful with it and protect it from toxins. The spirogyra does not contain harmful substances itself but helps the body to excrete them. Initially, this can cause symptoms as a healing response. See also section: What reactions can occur?

- Spirulina excretes chemicals, heavy metals, and radiation substances and regenerates the detox and elimination organs: skin, intestines, lungs, liver and kidneys.
- The algae reduce the side effects of drugs.

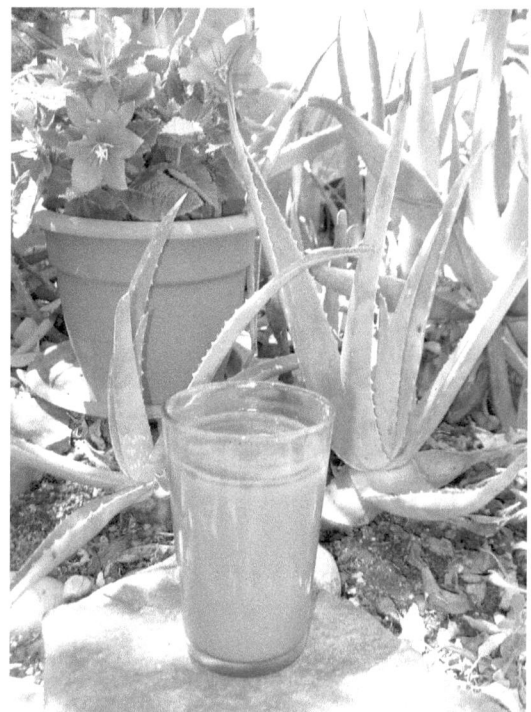

II. FASTING CURE, ENERGIZING & PERSONALITY FORMING

Spirulina fasting for a basic milieu

If you want to get and stay healthy, it is necessary to rid the body of toxins (acids) to create an alkaline environment and to support the natural cellular respiration! Once the body is alkaline and rich in oxygen, every disease stops even cancer. For this realization, the Swedish Karolinska Institute awarded Dr. Otto Heinrich Warburg in 1931 the Nobel Prize in Medicine. It is clear why the conventional medicine ignores this fact: The cancer Mafia or the medical-scientific establishment do not want to give up their multi-million deals. One oncologist alone can ensure a pharmacist's annual turnover of around €6,000,000 says the physician Ulrich Fritz.

http://www.stern.de/investigativ/stern-recherche--die-skrupellosen-geschaefte-der-krebsmafia-6692272.html

http://www.theforbiddenknowledge.com/hardtruth/cancer_business.htm

If when turning over your problems you can not get a restful sleep, treat yourself every evening with an alkaline drink and learn about the positive effect of a basic condition as my husband did on July 4, 2016. Every night Peter used to drink one or two bottles of red wine since supposedly he could hardly sleep without it. But on July 2, he did risk a look at the scale. Having digested the shock of his disastrous weight balance, he changed from wine to water. Especially, since he had after the enjoyment of wine, usually released his weaker self, indulging in his usual gormandize orgy. On the morning after the first night without the circling stimulating poisons, he complained of insomnia. Next evening I gave him a glass of water with 1 teaspoon of organic sulfur (MSM or methylsulfonylmethane), ½ teaspoon magnesium citrate and a pinch of borax. These mineral salts I used on my sulfur cure from the book *WATER CONNECTS THE WORLDS*, chapter water activation and dietary supplements for radiantly healthy people, animals, and plants. Next morning I was greeted by a beaming man: I've slept through til 7. Since then the minerals belong to our program which also seems to stimulate physical activity. If you want to lose weight, keep in mind: an acidic milieu complicates the fat reduction.

But now let's get to the Spirulina fasting. Consistently my readers express their positive experiences consuming Spirulina during fasting. You feel excellent with the algae even after several days. Formerly when fasting without Spirulina, they were hungry and without energy because the microorganism can cure the lack of nutrients during fasting with incredibly few calories. When fasting, you feel best when your intestines are clean. If you want to lose weight without negative health effects, the alga is ideal. Since it contains 60% protein, you will never have more energy in your live as in these days. Your body can recover and repair at rest because Spirulina is particularly easy to digest. I feel best when juice fasting with Spirulina. It is a practical method, especially for professionals. For a fast food mix some apple juice, applesauce, banana or vegetables with a little water and 1 tablespoon Spirulina powder in a blender (see recipe section). The smoothies detoxify and purify. They help all cells to regenerate. The high protein content in Spirulina causes the thyroid to boost the metabolism melting the fat stores. Spirulina's uncountable nutrients plus the freshly squeezed juices from fruits and vegetables deliver valuable enzymes, vitamins, and minerals.

The US businessman and author Norman W. Walker was an advocate of fresh juice cures. He enjoyed freshly squeezed juices and ascribed to them his advanced age of 99 years. He may have become well over 100 if he had not died as a result of an accident.

In addition to Spirulina, you can deacidify the cells with spring plants such as nettle, wild garlic, coriander, cleavers, dandelion, and plantain. Also, basic mineral supplements are suitable for cleaning the cells. Your body is entirely clean when your sweat and your urine smell after your last enjoyed fruit.

Colon and liver cleansing: a guarantee for well-being and healing

A clean intestine is a requirement for the optimal absorption of Spirulina agents. Also, if you feel sick and nothing seems to help you can clean your colon with Epsom salt, psyllium husk powder or enemas. For that you drink in the first week every morning 1 teaspoon Epsom salts (magnesium sulfate) dissolved in ¼ liter of water, half an hour before breakfast. In the 2nd week, every 2nd morning then only twice a week and finally once. After four weeks the intestine should be cleaned, and you can use the blue-green microalgae. Then treat your gut and even more your liver with some coffee enemas. The coffee enema is part of the Gerson cancer diet which the raw food pioneer Dr. Max Gerson developed after World War II. But only Prince Charles made it known worldwide by recognizing publicly daily coffee enemas as an effective anticancer agent.

Coffee enemas help the liver with its detoxification function. It can thus dispose of more toxins from the human organism in the gut. Because the bitter coffee enhances the bile ducts, stimulates bile production and releases the pollutants from the bile ducts of the liver. Thus the capacity of the liver improves. It can filter poisons and metabolic wastes now effectively, ensuring pure blood. Impaired liver function can cause enormous damage to your health. If you suffer from allergy, drowsiness, intestinal cramps, depression, diarrhea, stomach ailments, migraine or fatigue, a coffee enema can rapidly eliminate your symptoms. Here's how to make it:

Bring 1 liter of water to a boil, add 2-3 tbsp organic coffee, allow to cook for 3 minutes then let it steep 15 minutes. Bring 1 liter of water to a boil, add 2-3 tbsp organic coffee, allow to cook for 3 minutes then let it steep 15 minutes. Pour the coffee through a fine sieve. Allow to cool it down to body temperature. Insert it rectally with an enema bag or a Klyso Klistier Irrigator. With this pump, gently insert the liquid with self-regulated pressure into the intestine. Hold the coffee no longer than 15 minutes and no less than 10.

To increase the lactobacilli and calm the possibly irritable bowel helps a rectal implant with 1 tsp Spirulina, 1 tbsp aloe vera juice and 1 cup of water shaken in a screw top jar. You can also use 10 drops of 25% dextrorotatory lactic acid drops and Spirulina. These colonize the intestine with the new beneficial microorganisms. Sheep yogurt and, in moderation lactate vegetables also can restore the intestine. To stimulate the intestinal peristalsis, you can daily perform a gentle massage of the intestine. A drink with psyllium husk powder (PHP) in the evening brings a pleasant excretion. If you don't like Epsom salts, you can also use PHP for a colon cleansing: For 4 weeks in the morning, 1½ hours before breakfast, between meals and 1½ hours after dinner or before bedtime stir 1 tablespoon PHP in ¼ liter of liquid and drink it promptly or eat it 10 minutes later as porridge. After that, drink plenty of water.

Mitochondrial energy medicine

Recently my fellow author Wolfgang Meyer made me aware of his experience with energy and regulatory medicine. This method is based on Space Medicine. The following video contains a lecture of Prof. Dr. Enrico Edinger. Though you may not understand German, you should see the amazing before and after pictures of the young woman whose face cells grew completely back to normal within two and a half months after a serious car accident (page 47).

http://www.inakarb.de/wp-content/uploads/2015/08/behandlungserfolge_und_technische_systeme.pdf

The following link leads you to information in your language by Dr. Mark Sircus, a disputed acupuncturist, and doctor of oriental and pastoral medicine:

http://drsircus.com/medicine/mitochondrial-medicine-cocktails/

But in connection with Spirulina, it is more of interest that over 90% diseases are caused by an imbalance of the autonomic nervous system. Edinger thinks they have triggered by an adrenaline deficiency showing through fatigue, dizziness, listlessness, and difficulty in concentrating. The stress hormone is produced in the adrenal medulla and supplies energy, oxygen intake, and fat loss. It regulates blood circulation and digestion, increases the heart rate and blood pressure and reduces sensitivity to pain. So if you want to get rid of typical burnout symptoms and overweight, Spirulina is a true wonder weapon. Because it contains everything in the natural state which is necessary for the formation of adrenalin: tyrosine, phenylalanine, vitamin C, vitamin B6, magnesium, folic acid, copper ...

The cornucopia of vital substances in the blue-green algae regulate and harmonize all metabolic processes in the body: liver and bowel function, insulin level, water balance, fat metabolism, hunger, pH, bloodstream ...

Synthetic multivitamins are known to cause side effects. Therefore and due to our food void of vital substances, I can only recommend taking an excellent Spirulina brand every day. My heavy smoking girlfriend is the best proof. She takes the algae daily for nearly 20 years. Her two sisters are non-smoking. The elder suffers from kidney failure the younger from rheumatism. They both think it's unfair but want to know nothing of Spirulina. Or loosely based on Goethe: I hear the message well, but lack faith.

Into a new era of love and light

There is a land of the living and a land of the dead, and the bridge is love, the only survival, the only meaning.

Thornton Wilde

Reading the title of this book, you may have wondered what it is all about with the new era. On December 31, 2012, ended a 400-year continuous cycle of the Mayan calendar. With it, according to Felipe Gomez of the Maya alliance Oxlaljuj Ajpop, would begin a new period, accompanied by changes in personal, family and community level, leading to harmony and balance between man and nature.

http://phys.org/news/2012-10-maya-demand-doomsday-myth.html

In 1950, the book "The Last Day" of the German author Paul Otto Hesse came out. There we learned for the first time about the Photon Belt and the accompanying manasic radiation. At the end of the 80s, I read in various esoteric books about this phenomenon. Just as the earth rotates around the sun in 365 days, the sun and its planets are supposed to circle in 25,860 years around the Central Sun Alcyone in the Pleiades constellation. In this orbit, we should twice have 2000 years of light and love after 10,500 years of darkness. The sages of antiquity marked these periods as the golden age. Such a light Age of Christ Consciousness would be lying ahead. Some say we are already in it.

With all the power-hunger, brutality, and corruption of cold-hearted rulers, the fraud and greed of bankers and industry executives doubts are indicated. Also on the concept of separating the wheat from the chaff, the question should be allowed: Who decides on useful and useless?

https://en.wikipedia.org/wiki/Photon_belt

I can hardly promise you that we are in for a golden age. But if the people would finally realize that we are all one whether black, white, red, yellow, rich or poor, that might be a start. The next link leads you to the video Raw Footage of Michael Tellinger. He provides evidence that all humans were cloned in South Africa. So why the racial conflicts?

https://www.youtube.com/watch?v=yHu1x0k8T-0

The esoteric should be classified as a frontier science just as highly as the sparsely documented string theory. This implies: Particles are no more particles, but only so-called vibrations of the space-time.

https://en.wikipedia.org/wiki/String_theory

It can be seen from this that the transitions between science and outsider theories are fluid. In my book *How Water Connects Our WORLDS*, I introduce new equally undefined energy technologies and their inventors. These are tangible evidence of the existence of spirit. And if something works, it can not violate the laws of physics. Quantum physicists have indeed proved that the world of action and substance is energy or spirit. Every feeling, every thought, every word and deed are energy. What we think, feel, speak or write is the seed in the field of our life. The years of light we can enjoy when the greedy few stop grasping for short-term profits and realize that they have to live at the end with the damage caused by themselves and if they become aware that reincarnation and karma are no esoteric blah. I suggest reading Dethlefsen's Book *The Challenge of Fate*, in which he explains the esoteric as an unscientific way of looking at the reality. Or, if you like it more entertaining you can read my autobiographical novel *Family Code*. The reincarnation serves the perfection of the soul linking with the law noted by Paul in the Galatians: You reap what you sow. Jesus explained past incarnations like this: "When you see your likeness, you rejoice. But when you see your images which came into being before you, and which neither die nor become manifest, how much you will have to bear!" (Gospel of Thomas, verse 84).

Today we term the universal law of cause and effect: karma strikes back. Under this law, there is no guilt we can pin on somebody. There is also no accident and no luck. There is only cause and effect which can be many centuries and incarnations apart. Luck, bad luck, and chance only show the unrecognized law. I wish you that you will make the knowledge available that's always been there. And I wish all of us that we can live in love, freedom, unity and dignity which is to have proper housing, clothing, and feeding. This would be possible if the greedy few would allow converting space energy into electrical energy what Nikola Tesla already had done about 100 years ago. There are also cars running with water, but the oil magnates have their way to bribe, threaten, and even kill the inventors in case the bribing and threatening didn't work out. About this, you can read in my above-mentioned water book. We better contact our elected officials and ask for free energy.

Every fall, the Jupiter-Verlag organizes the International Free Energy Congress. So you can convince yourself that the paradigm shift in the energy supply is impending.

The Jupiter-Verlag also publishes the NET-Journal, the only German-language magazine dealing with unconventional energy technologies.

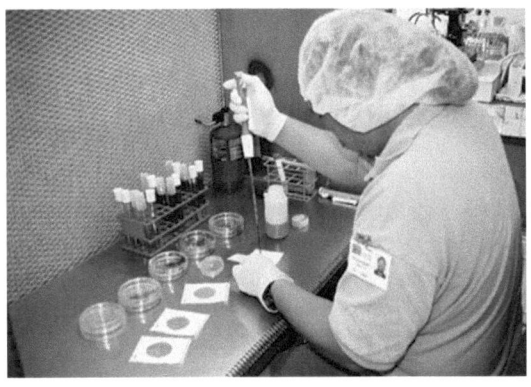

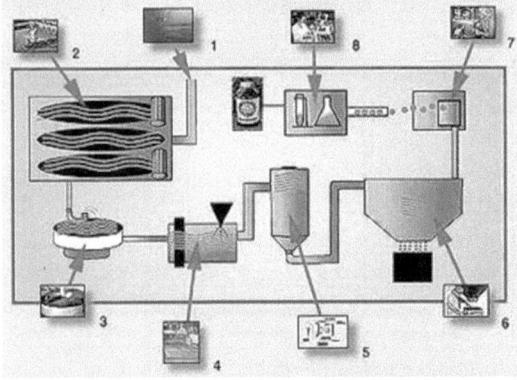

1. Deepwater resource
2. Breeding ponds
3. Separation sections
4. Vacuum-washing system
5. Ocean-cold drying
6. Finished powder
7. Cold compression tabletting
8. Extensive quality analysis

III. SPIRULINA PLATENSIS

What is Spirulina?

If you have come to appreciate the promising microorganism you may want to look at it more closely:

Scientific classifikation of Spirulina

Domain	Bacteria
Kingdom	Eubacteria
Phylum	Cyanobacteria
Order	Spirulinales
Family	Spirul inaceae
Genus	Spirulina

Turpin ex Gomont 1892

The correct name of the blue-green alga is Arthrospira platensis. But because of historic reasons, it is usually referred to as Spirulina platensis. On warm alkaline lakes of subtropical latitudes, the twisted threads form a fluorescent blue-green carpet in the sunlight serving fish and birds as main food. The charming flamingos living in the area of East African soda lakes owe Spirulina their pink color. The 4 % carotenoids in Spirulina, responsible for this, are covered by the blue pigment phycocyanin and the green chlorophyll. On the cusp of plant and animal, the cyanobacteria are placed a little higher than the plant as they have neither a true nucleus nor plant-typical hard cell walls. The unicellular organisms need sunlight for using the organic carbon. The greater the exposure to light the faster and larger they grow. The cylindrical cells are up to a millimeter in size and can be seen with the naked eye. They reproduce asexually by simple constriction of the threads, so by simple cell division without DNA duplication. The chlorophyll in Spirulina is the same as the one in plants only it is distributed throughout

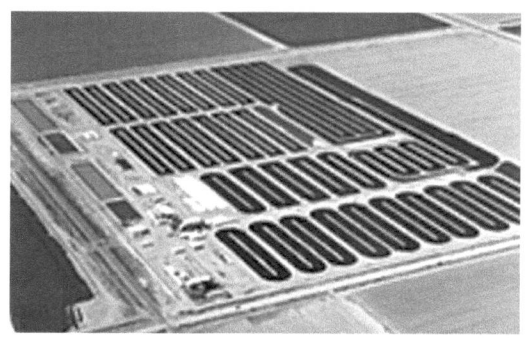

the cell and not limited as with greenery only to the chloroplast. Spirulina grows best in very warm alkaline lakes of 35 to 40°C with a salinity of 15 to 20% (seawater contains 3%) and a pH-value of 8-11. For other organisms, this environment is too salty and too hot. This allows Spirulina to maintain hygienic conditions, one reason why cyanobacteria could survive from early times until today. They withstand next to extreme temperatures also radioactivity. Though they hardly grow under extreme conditions, life continues. In a cold environment, Spirulina looks like worms, in the heat, they turn like screws. They react inversely to us. We pull ourselves together when we are cold and stretch in the warm sun. We need the oxygen the algae release and the algae need the CO2 we exhale. Solidly coiled they multiply fastest and double their biomass in 2 to 5 days. Thus it would be easy to build saltwater pools in any place in the Third World and to put an end to world hunger!

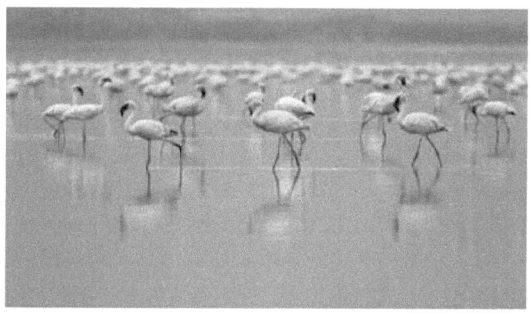

Even in our latitudes with solar or better space energy heated Spirulina ponds could everywhere provide for food and better CO2 conditions of the air we breathe.

History of the oldest foodstuff

About 3.6 billion years ago, the cyanobacteria should have started to create the oxygen atmosphere of our planet. Their blue pigment evidently represents the common origin of plant and animal life, including humans. Because the molecular structure of this phytochemical contains both magnesium and iron they thus precede the chlorophyll and hemoglobin. Spirulina contains 15% of this phytochemical.

Precursors of Spirulina platensis split water molecules with the help of sunlight to produce food from the surrounding minerals and gasses: they processed carbon dioxide (CO2) to carbohydrates, amino acids and nitrogen to protein. In this process of food production, they released oxygen, thus creating a life-friendly uniformly ordered whole. So blue-green algae form a recycling system with humans and other aerobe. As already mentioned, animals dependent on oxygen need oxygen and release CO2into the atmosphere!

The Maya and Aztecs of ancient Central America appreciated the strengthening and regenerating effect of Spirulina and used it daily in their diet. With baskets, they scooped the green slag foam from the shallow Lake Chad. Some Spirulina researchers believe that the lichen-forming crusts of rocks and soil is the manna mentioned in the Bible. God should have given this symbiosis of fungus and blue-green algae the Israelis when they starved in the desert. History provides two dozens more concrete examples of the protein and vital substance source used in soups, sauces or as spread:

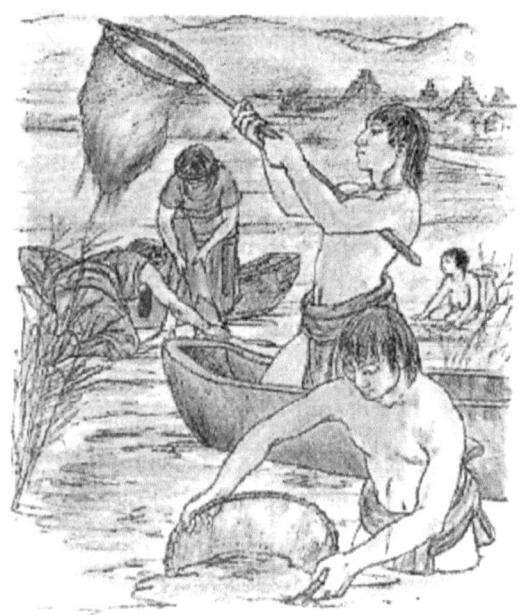

When in 1521 the Spanish conquistadors invaded the Aztec empire (Mexico), Bernal Diaz del Castillo, a member of the troops of Hernán Cortés, observed that the natives subsisted on pulpy masses, corn, beans, and a green substance. They called it tecuitlatl and ascribed to it a mysterious, healing and strengthening effect.

In 1827, J. P. Turpin isolated the cyanobacteria, and Lothar Geitler classified it. But only in 1940 reported the phycologist Pierre-Augustin Dangeard and 1964 the botanist Jean Leonhard on the practices of the Kanembu folks: They scooped the strange blue-green foam from the surface of Lake Chad and let it dry into cakes. In 1967, Hiroshi Nakamura took notice of the French National Petroleum Center's Spirulina projects. He had long been interested in algae as a protein source for the starving world and therefore was enthusiastic about the variety of uses of this particularly high-quality type. Nakamura, his Japanese team and his American colleague Christopher Hills were pioneers in the Spirulina research. As mentioned, the Japanese are world leaders in the consumption of the Green Gold and therefore probably live longer than residents of other industrialized nations. After all, there were Frisian bakers who started baking hearty Spirulina rolls that sold like hotcakes.

• The life of plants and animals has probably evolved from the blue pigment phycocyanin.

• The cyanobacteria produced the first food via photosynthesis: from carbon carbohydrates, and from amino acids and nitrogen protein.

• Cyanobacteria require CO2 and release oxygen. They form a recycling system with oxygen-dependent organisms.

• The survival from the Precambrian till today the microorganisms owe their tolerance to extreme temperatures, high salinity, toxic gasses and radioactive radiation.

• The Maya and Aztecs used Spirulina in maize and bean dishes for strengthening and regeneration.

• In 1827 discovered and named by a German, the microalgae attracted attention only 140 years later.

• Hiroshi Nakamura and Christopher Hill are the pioneers of Spirulina research.

Visions and necessity

As intelligent beings, we see it as our task to set in motion creative processes in our plane of existence. Thereby we receive help from so-called coincidences. Creating our heaven on earth we have heavenly assistance in problem-solving and, therefore, we activate creation processes. If we ask for a future in which all creatures can breathe clean air, live in decent homes and do not go hungry we meet a general need. If we act according to our spiritual gifts instead of wasting our vigor to fight against something we save time, money and energy. We better use the healing, cleansing, and beautification products of nature rather than contaminate our groundwater via sewage with household chemicals, cosmetics, and medicines. If we want to protect our environment, we better make use of our power as consumers. We can call on preexisting space energy converters and support environmentally friendly and humanly managed companies. We have to focus on better prospects. With free energy, no nation would run after other nation's resources. No government would wage war for resources or terrorize, occupy and exploit other countries. We can all contribute to the creation of a better future!

Spirulina dreams to come true ASAP

• In villages of poor countries, space energy converter provide power for Spirulina farms for residents to have enough to eat and to get essential nutrients.

• Doctors prescribe according to Hippocrates Spirulina and other food remedies to improve health.

• In kindergartens and daycare centers, there are often delicious Spirulina dishes served hence hyperactive or depressive kids are rare.

• In retirement and nursing homes, the residents are dosed with the Green Gold daily to strengthen their immune system and nerves.

• For balancing a lack of nutrients, Spirulina powder is added to many foods.

• Fast food restaurants outdo each other with tasty lentil, bean and veggie burgers containing Spirulina.

• Due to Spirulina as fodder addition, the drug use for livestock and animals ready for slaughter is reduced.

• Spirulina serves as hydrogen supplier for fuel cells. The lipids fed by industrial exhaust fumes are converted with methanol to biodiesel, not increasing the price of food.

• Spirulina powered biogas plants provide homes with energy and make us independent from the multinationals. Nuclear power plants are needless. No more oil from leaking wells and rusty tankers contaminate our oceans.

• Globally Spirulina cultures transform, e. g., in airlift reactors, organic waste matter into valuable biomass, such as food, pet food, remedies, and fuel.

• We transform disparaging thoughts into positive ones and oppressive regimes in democracies. All people act on the welfare of all living things.

• The alga's active components are used to manufacture most drugs.

• Their calming properties make Spirulina the wonder pill of our Brave New World.

Usage diversity of Spirulina in overview

- For the elimination of world hunger and to prevent child mortality and blindness due to vitamin A deficiency
- As a dietary supplement for the prevention of diseases
- As a food additive for domestic, agricultural and breeding animals and to intensify the color of fish and exotic birds
- As natural food colors serve the extracted blue and green pigments phycocyanin and chlorophyll
- As easy to be stored means of survival in times of crisis
- In space programs of the NASA: as food for astronauts, for air purification and conversion of waste and excreta
- For natural fertilization of useful and ornamental plants
- For manufacturing organic plastic bags

http://algix.com/from-plastic-pollution-to-an-algae-solution/

- As natural cosmetics to improve skin structure (e. g., with water for masks or as an additive in cellulite or facial creams)
- As biofuel

http://energy.gov/eere/videos/energy-101-algae-fuel

Microalgae breeding by chance

In the Mid-1940s, some workers in the production of soda ash on Lake Texcoco north of Mexico City discovered the Spirulina cultivation by accident. They set up a spare pool and filled it with salt enriched water. There the algae grew lusher than on the lake. So they get on to the track of the Spirulina cultivation. Now the Texcoco Lake is dry. The famous lakes in which today flourish 35 types of Spirulina are the Lake Chad in central Africa, the Kenyan lakes Nakuru and Turkana and the Aranguadi lake in Ethiopia. The cultures from these lakes are kept in glass containers and transported when needed in food grade plastic lined pools. Since the 1960s, the production of algae increases substantially. More and more people discover the advantage of this dietary supplement. Among the most prolific breeders are the farmers on Hawaii, Hainan, Taiwan and in Southern California. There the Spirulina cultures as usual at the farms are gently mixed by paddle wheels.

In the Andes, the growers cultivate in shallow water via an inclined plane. In a modern algae production plant in the Altmark's Klötze, the microorganisms thrive in kilometer-long glass tubes, in Lower Saxony in Bassum in incubator tubes. Worldwide Spirulina farmers produce over 12,000 tons of dry matter per year. Beginning of this century the production was less than 5,000 t.

If you want to cultivate Spirulina in agriculture or at home, Jean-Paul Jourdan's detailed manual can help you. He describes the different scales of the cyanobacteria production under different physical and climatic conditions. JPJ developed smaller projects of Spirulina breeding in Europe and Africa.

antenna.ch/en/documents/Jourdan_UK.pdf

Jourdan explains the big quality differences in as much as some Asian companies extract phycocyanin and sell it to food producers as a food coloring. The robbed rest they offer cheaper to be competitive on the world market. Therefore Jourdan advocates the labeling of the phycocyanin content. Please ask for an analysis!

www.berrysmith.org/news/spirulina-expert-jean-paul-jourdan

The following links show small Spirulina production facilities. Maybe you also would like to be self-sufficient with such a mini-farm.

www.smartmicrofarms.com/slideshows/olympia-microfarm/

www.spirulinasource.co

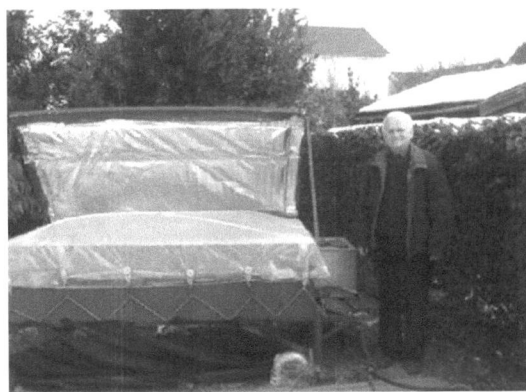

The water in which the cultures flourish contains primarily soda (sodium carbonate), nitrogen, phosphorus, iron and other minerals and trace elements. The cultures are fertilized with various minerals. Next to J.P. Jourdan there are some hundred other Spirulina growers in southern France. It is also a Frenchman who succeeded in producing 100% biodegradable plastic granules from seaweed.

http://www.algopack.com/algopackgb.php

You can also help a couple with their Spirulina project in Monchique, Portugal. Cristina and George propose a stay under a tent with hot water, shower, and wifi. They expect you to work there for 5 hours a day 5 days a week. You will learn to grow Spirulina and be able to reproduce the project on the various unused Portuguese land. See also page 48.

spirulina-da-serra.com/contact-spirulina-da-serra

The conventional medicine as well as pharmaceutical companies, their lobbyists, and trolls like to mix up Spirulina platensis with the equally blue-green alga Aphanizomenon flosaque (AFA). AFA grows in the Klamath Lake in Oregon. By contrast, Spirulina grows to maximize hygienic in food-grade plastic lined pools. So they are contrary to the AFA algae protected against microcystins and other contaminants. As the Spirulina cultures on the Hawaiian Big Island, the AFA cultures are fertilized with minerals and trace elements from volcanic rocks. The consumers of blue-green algae known to me take both types, Spirulina daily and AFA as a cure when they need more energy (Simonson 2000).

Bringing in the harvest

With favorable weather conditions, the workers harvest weekly. In the individual basins, they mix in turn the cultures. Since there is only one filter system, they pump out the pools one after the other but only to two-thirds. The rest of the cultures remains for propagating the next generation. The collected water flows back into the pools. The paper-thin spiral threads are filtered with fine mesh screens of stainless steel. When harvesting with steel nets, the workers clean the algae several times with fresh water and afterward concentrate it with vibrating sieves.

The dehydration process

Previously Spirulina was freeze-dried and long exposed to oxygen, resulting in a loss of quality. Today large Spirulina producers usually dry the culture in the spray dryer. Then they filter it with lattice screens and put the collected algae mass on vibrating sieves where they get further concentrated. Finally, the workers dehydrate the concentrate further on a vacuum feeder band filter. The algae powder coming out of the dryer is immediately vacuum packed and taken to the shipping.

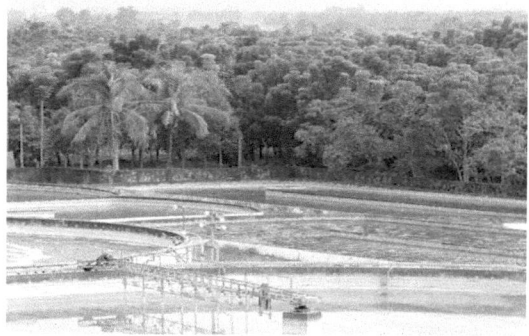

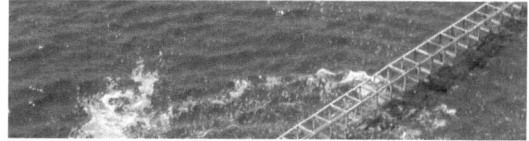

The pressing of the tablets

In producing the tablets are huge differences in quality. Often powders are mixed with cheap binders, on high-speed machines compressed in molds and hot ejected. Or before ejecting the producers stir in granules. Thus the algae concentrate is subjected to prolonged exposure to oxygen. In such processes, we have to reckon with a loss of up to half of the carotene content. So you better buy powder instead of any cheap tablets or best pay attention to quality.

• 35 species of Spirulina grow in salt-lakes of subtropical latitudes. From there the crops grown in ponds originate.

• The cultures usually become enriched with various minerals.

- Slow air drying conserves heat-labile vital substances.
- Spirulina of optimum quality is pleasant in flavor.
- Cheap compressed tablets contain few vital substances.

How to take Spirulina

If you take Spirulina as a food supplement, 3 x 2 tablets daily are enough.

To reduce weight, replace at least one meal with a Spirulina drink from the recipe section with 1 tablespoon of powder. You can also stir 1 tbsp in applesauce or fruit or vegetable juice. If you want to gain or keep your weight, take your ration after the meal. If you are neither evidently ill nor feel quite healthy because you may suffer from a difficult to detect deficiency syndrome, with 20 tablets or 2 teaspoons of algae powder per day you can attain nutritional harmony, vitality, and performance again. If you are ill and want to prove Spirulina's healing benefits you can take 3 heaped teaspoons to tablespoons of powder or 30 to 60 tablets daily. Whether you take the algae concentrate in powder form or as tablets is up to you. It is best to consume it in 1 to 2 servings as a snack. I mix the flour with the same amount of grated almonds, coconuts or Chufanutlets since it better connects with liquids. Of this, I take 1 to 2 tablespoons with apricot or apple juice. Important: If you suffer from pain, depression, diabetes or high blood pressure, it would be better to consume the algae distributed throughout the day. If you tend to forget taking tabs, you better use the green flour in juice, broth or porridge. Your hunger will always be a reminder to consume an avocado, a broth or fruit puree with algae powder. As beverage additive or forced into a banana the preparation of these delicious snacks is almost as fast as filling a water glass and counting the tablets. Because of possibly new insights regarding blocking vitamin B12 analogs, you better don't combine Spirulina all too often with another vitamin B12-containing food.

If you become reminded by signs of illness because the body is missing something, e. g., when you have headaches, your eyes burn, or the throat hurts, you take some tablets with water. If you suck them, Spirulina's active ingredients mixed with the saliva get very quickly through the oral mucosa into the blood. My allergic reaction to cat hair is gone this way after 3 to 4 minutes.

- As a dietary supplement with a balanced diet take 3 x 2 tablets or 3 x ¼ tsp powder. With a one-sided diet take the double or triple amount.
- To reduce weight, take 9-14 tablets or 1 teaspoon powder 1 hour before the main meals with ½ liter of fluid.
- If you feel unwell, take 20 Spirulina tabs or 2 teaspoon algae flour per day.
- With illness take 3 teaspoons up to 3 tablespoons powder or 30-60 tablets daily.

What reactions can occur?

Spirulina is a natural food supplement, no chemical preparation. Possible side effects of the algae are therefore generally of positive nature: they show the excretion of toxins. That could cause discomfort. Therefore it is advisable that you slowly get used to the vital substance bomb. Due to the high cleansing effect, it may initially lead to bloating, intestinal winds, diarrhea, or dizziness. Then you better take a half tablet 3 times a day in the first three days and increase the dose every three days by a half. To promote the detoxification process, drink daily 6 to 8 glasses of pure non-carbonated water. (Meyer 2016)

Initially, you may have no side effects. After a few weeks, reactions usually occur because taking daily 3 or more tabs for 4 to 6 weeks builds up the body's defenses. The now invigorated white blood cells launch a blow against aggressive foreign bodies and germs, polluting the blood. The antibodies of this antigen-antibody reaction (immune complexes) must be eliminated. Otherwise, you may develop immune complex diseases. So better drink lots of pure water. You best acquire a good device to improve your tap water and enjoy it as a personalized spring water. This defensive battle is not always smooth and unnoticed. You may have reactions. Mentally you feel fit. But you may frequently eliminate, sweat and cough. The nose may run, and the throat may feel rough. But these reactions are healing signs. If you don't understand this mechanism, you could despite all the initial enthusiasm about Spirulina's positive effects say, that stuff does not help in the long run because I caught a cold again. Now you better hang on since this is a normal reaction to the initiated cleansing process. It usually occurs after 4 to 6 weeks and can be eased with grapefruit seed extract, H2O2, silver ions (CS), cranberries, papaya, pineapple, lapacho tea and plenty of pure water.

According to Hering's Law, all healing comes first from the inside out. Symptoms such as swelling of lymph nodes, fever, runny nose, cough, and sputum are natural reactions of cleaning the body.

Upon completion of this elimination phase, it may still come to such reactions up to three times at intervals of 4-6 weeks depending on the degree of poisoning of the body. During the next phase of detoxing the body is freed of metabolic waste. Colon cleansing, fasting, enemas and sauna sessions assist the detox. The following two cleansing phases stimulate the cellular metabolism, increase the energy level and repair the cells.

• With cleansing reactions such as bloating or diarrhea start with 3 x ½ tabs and increase the dose every 3 days by a ½.

• 3-4 times in each case after 4-6 weeks positive excretion symptoms can occur: a runny nose, sore throat or a cough.

• After 4 to 6 months the immune system is completely rebuilt.

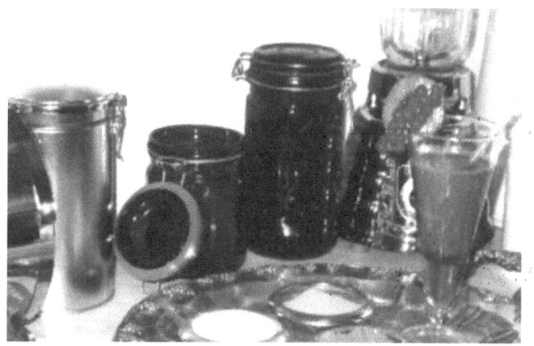

Proper storage protects nutrients and biophotons

Naturally grown foods are light bearers, so they carry the sun's energy within. To preserve the light energy, store Spirulina airtight in a dark place.

Probably, for this reason, even the ancient Egyptians used to preserve precious essences and remedies in violet, blue or golden containers because herbal extracts stay longer fresh and alive there. Improper storage can cause enormous energy loss. We better not waste our good money for valuable substances by closing the lid carelessly or select unsuitable containers.

IV. COMPONENTS OF SPIRULINA

Unique active agents of the blue-green microalgae

Spirulina contains between 60 and 70 percent of valuable, easily digestible protein. With no species-appropriate feeding and care of the animals used in our diet, the best vegetable protein gains in importance. For more than 30 years Spirulina is known to strengthen the immune system and to prevent cancer. Instead of performing more animal-excruciating studies it would be better except for the disease industry to supplement the food with Spirulina. It would protect us, our animal friends and the planet. Even the permanent tinkering on new health reforms would no longer be necessary.

Stored sunlight could be the true value of cyanobacteria, but the concentrated nutritional substances are also highly presentable. Following an overview of the pigments, polysaccharides, essential fatty acids, sulfolipids, glycolipids, vitamins and minerals in Spirulina.

Phycocyanin strengthens the immune system and detoxifies the body

The food industry uses the blue pigment of the algae as a natural colorant for drinks, sweets, chewing gums and desserts. It also acts as a free radical scavenger and as a powerful antioxidant. Independent studies confirm an anti-inflammatory effect of phycocyanin. It accelerates wound healing and helps in the cure of ulcers. Numerous studies show that phycocyanin possesses antiviral and anti-cancer properties. But how works the immunostimulatory pigment that we find only in blue-green algae? It increases the activity of lymphocytes and ensures proper cellular control functions. It inhibits the growth, proliferation and the formation of cancer, even the most dangerous pancreas cancer as discovered by Renata Koníčková and her fellow researchers from the Charles University in Prague. It was strange that a day after the son of my friend left his body, ravaged by metastatic pancreatic cancer, I again looked for the latest Spirulina studies to write a blog report. *The aim of the study was to evaluate the potential anticancer effects of Spirulina platensis and derived from the cyanobacterium tetrapyrrole in the experimental model of pancreatic cancer.* (2014)

The growth-inhibitory effect of Spirulina and its components phycocyanobilin (PCB) and chlorophyll were tested on several human pancreatic cancer cell lines and xenografted on nude mice, meaning, living from one to the other transmitted organism. The cancer cell growth inhibitory effect of Spirulina has thus been shown also on the living organism where it was proven already after the third day of treatment. The cancer cell growth inhibitory effect of Spirulina has thus been shown also on living organisms. The inhibition of pancreatic tumor growth was shown already after three days treatment. Spirulina or its tetrapyrrolic components significantly reduces the spread of experimental pancreatic cancer. So this edible alga is used for cancer prevention and may also improve liver dysfunction. http://www.marianne-e-meyer.com/2014/03/24/spirulina-hemmt-das-pankreas-krebswachstum/

Also in March 2014 the biophysicists M. Kaur Saini and S. Nath Sanyal of the Panjab University in Chandigarh, India, confirmed that the blue pigment in Spirulina is an effective natural supplement for the prevention of colon cancer. In 2008, Chen and Wong of the University of Hong Kong found out that the antioxidant activity of selenium-enriched phycocyanin (Se PC) was even stronger. It also showed protective effects on red blood cells against hydrogen peroxide (H2O2) caused damage to the genetic material. Se-PC also showed strong activity against melanoma and breast cancer cells. The researchers summed up: Selenium-enriched phycocyanin is a promising natural remedy for the prevention of cancer.

In 2009 the same researchers examined the anti-cancer potential of Se-PC and found that it inhibits the growth of breast cancer cells. Fukino and its Japanese research colleagues discovered: Phycocyanin prevents the poisoning of the kidneys and thus the failure of that organ.

We can assume that phycocyanin indicates the common origin of the life of plants and animals including men because the molecular structure comprises magnesium as in the plant cell and iron as in the animal or human cell. Phycocyanin is thus clearly the predecessor of chlorophyll and hemoglobin. Spirulina contains 12 to 15% Phycocyanin.

In 2007, Vadiraja and colleagues discovered that the blue pigment in Spirulina protects the liver among others from the harmful solvent medium carbon tetrachloride. Roy and colleagues from the University of Hyderabad also researched in 2007 the potential of phycocyanin. It induces programmed cell death of liver cancer cells. The Indian researchers pointed to a 50 % decrease in the proliferation of S-and R-HepG2 cells treated with 40 and 50 microns phycocyanin for 24 hours.

- The blue pigment in Spirulina detoxifies and protects the kidneys.

- Phycocyanin prevents heavy metal poisoning.
- The blue protein pigment inhibits pancreatic cancer 3 days after ingestion.

SOD, the anti-aging Enzyme

In 1968 the biochemist Irwin Fridovich and his colleagues at Duke University in North Carolina isolated for the first time the enzyme superoxide dismutase (SOD) as a destroyer of oxygen radical hydrogen peroxide (H2O2; Kotulak 1991).

This discovery was an important step forward in the longevity research. The body produces SOD to protect itself against damaging environmental influences. The more SOD we have, the longer we live. Our inner healer provides the substances to protect us from radicals, UV rays, radioactive substances, chemicals, gasses, drugs, heated fats, and oxygen. However, the organism must be supplied with the required micronutrients or biophotons for the making. Spirulina contains all the colors of the spectrum and all the nutrients needed by the body to produce this enzyme: zinc, copper, and manganese are the most important.

Whether the biophotons or the chemical elements in Spirulina bestow us radiant health, can be all the same to us. Biochemists and biophysicists like to argue whether cells are constructed by micronutrients or frequencies of light or color respectively. So we are well advised to provide us with sun-ripened fresh food. Since there are documented persons who do not eat it could be that the light keeps us alive. Although I have read Jasmuheen's books, I have not however verified it personally, but I know people who got along for months without food. Experiments with cell cultures and in living organisms have shown that SOD-protected tissue remains healthy while unprotected cultures develop cancer.

Studies on the activity of SOD in cancer cells have shown: In malignancy, the SOD levels are drastically reduced (Kugler 1994).

Since Spirulina contains this most powerful antioxidant it can protect us from the diseases of civilization. In 1991, Dr. Richard Passwater proved in clinical trials that SOD protects us against radioactivity. He conducted double-blind placebo-controlled tests on patients with bladder cancer undergoing radiotherapy and found out: SOD offers protection against ionizing radiation. Conventional medicine uses this enzyme, known as orgotein, as an anti-inflammatory agent. However, studies have shown: A diet with adequate amounts of copper, zinc, and manganese is preferable to taking SOD preparations. Because the SOD activity in tissues showed only with nutrient adequate food. The drug administration remained without any effect (loc. cit.). This confirms the biophoton research: Synthetic is not natural, as you can see in the corresponding chapter. This result athletes can take to heart who aim for a healthy muscle building.

Sports physicians from Taiwan tested the preventive effect of Spirulina on muscle damage caused by exercise-induced oxidative stress. For 3 weeks, 16 students took Spirulina in addition to their regular diet. The results of the blood tests showed that the supplementation with Spirulina increased the activity of superoxide dismutase significantly. The study suggests that the consumption of the blue-green algae prevents musculoskeletal damage and reduces the exhaustion time (Lu et al. 2006).

Additional leprechauns in action

Other than SOD many enzymes act as biocatalysts. They regulate as a spark all metabolic processes and all the other physical processes which they make possible in the first place.

Without the biocatalysts formerly known as ferments, we could not think or breathe or digest. The fewer enzymes we eat, the less work for the metabolism. Enzymes help with inflammation, bruises, sprains, and arthritis. They dissolve immune complexes (antigen-antibody reaction) resulting from the defensive struggle of white blood cells with invading foreign bodies.

In an interview on May 22, 2000, Professor Dr. Günter Kahl from the Johann Wolfgang Goethe University in Frankfurt told me: Humans have about 100,000 genes, bacteria on the other hand only 2000 (Haemophilus influenzae) up to 3000 maximum. As a cyanobacterium, Spirulina has about 3000 genes roughly 2000 protein-coding genes, some are structural proteins, another part regulatory proteins. So you can expect about 1000-1500 enzymes. In reality, however, there are much more enzymes in the cell. On the one hand, there is more than one enzyme for the same reaction in the metabolism (so-called isoenzymes), on the other hand, the enzymes are often chemically modified before: about by introductions of phosphor or acetyl groups, to name just two.

• SOD rejuvenates and prolongs life. Spirulina contains SOD and all trace elements for the synthesizing.

• SOD protects against poisoning, radiation damage and other radicals.

• Cancer patients have low SOD levels.

• Food with SOD synthesizing minerals copper, zinc, and manganese (vegetables, mushrooms, oatmeal, whole wheat flour, fish, seeds, nuts, legumes) inhibit inflammation better than the synthetic orgotein.

• Spirulina has about 2000 protein-coding genes and about 1000-1500 enzymes.

Spirulina contains active vitamin B12

Vegetarians, vegans, frequent meat eaters, the elderly, alcoholics and persons with chronic digestive diseases may suffer from vitamin B12 deficiency manifesting by anemia (pallor, fatigue) or neurologic and psychiatric symptoms such as tingling, numbness, weakness, irritability, depression, and psychosis.

Popular science authors on nutrition write: Only animal foods contain vitamin B12 (cobalamin) leading to uncertainty among vegans. Vitamin B12 is generally obtained from the microbial production level. Therefore also the cyanobacterium Spirulina contains it, approximately as much as in calf's liver. The chanterelle and the black trumpet mushrooms contain 1-2.5 µg vitamin B12 per 100g of dry matter. Traces of B12 are in nori, wakame, miso and other eatable algae and fermented soy products. Plants growing on humus-rich soil can also contain traces of the hematopoietic vitamin as no or only slightly washed wild herbs from zero-emission zones. In grains not dead-sprayed with pesticides live tiny beetles and insects including the only water-soluble vitamin stored in the body. If you still fear to lack it, you can take vitamin 12 sublingual lozenges or drops, best as methylcobalamin. You can also inject vitamin B12.

However, most people with a Vitamin B12 deficiency should be carnivores, sweet tooth and the elderly. Because today's amounts of meat and sweets consumption lead to acidification, harming the stomach and the intestinal mucous membranes. It reduces the intrinsic factor and grinds down the protective coating of the nerve cells. Thus the vitamin B12 in food may eventually no longer be assimilated.

There are two forms of vitamin B12, the metabolically active which the body can absorb and use and the alleged harmful vitamin B12 analogs. Both forms are in Spirulina as well as in animal products. According to studies the pseudo-B12 vitamins hamper the metabolically active ones. Other tests refute this and others have shown that the vitamin B12 analogs do not impede the active ones only in raw-foodists.

Other researchers found the fresh alga to contain true vitamin B12, the dried one vitamin B12 analogs (Yamada 1999). The plant processes during drying seem to lead to chemical reactions that break down the vitamin B12. So if you want to grow Spirulina yourself as many southerners, you can consume the microorganisms immediately after harvesting. Less effort would be taking lozenges or drops keeping 5-10 secs in the mouth for the cobalamin to be absorbed through the oral mucosa. Since with an encrusted bowel swallowed pills are hardly of any use. Methylcobalamin can directly be used and does not have to be converted such as cyanocobalamin. It is, therefore, as well as the hydroxocobalamin ampoules the better choice.

Beta-carotene as cancer prophylaxis

Spirulina contains a varied selection of immune-strengthening carotenoids and more of the antioxidant beta-carotene than any other plant. Chinese researchers found that a beta-carotene extract inhibits the oxidative degradation of lipids and lowers blood glucose levels (Ma et al. 2016).

Studies from around the globe indicate that the consumption of carotene-rich fruits and vegetables reduces the risk of developing different types of cancer. But you should be warned about synthetic carotene supplements! Because the participants of studies in USA and Norway who ingested isolated carotene supplements had a higher risk of cancer. By contrast, it declined by 40% after eating only one carrot per day. In addition to the cancer-protection, beta-carotene ensures a healthy skin and prevents eye and cardiovascular diseases.

Chlorophyll detoxifies and cleanses the blood

The phytonutrient cleanses and detoxifies our vital juices. As mentioned above, the so-called green blood differs from the red blood pigment hemoglobin only by its magnesium core. The latter gives the chlorophyll the green color. Hemoglobin gets the red color from the iron core. This similarity with the red blood pigment is one of the reasons for the alga's positive effect on anemia because it makes a conversion from chlorophyll to hemoglobin possible.

Next to the formation of hemoglobin chlorophyll acts stimulating, kills hostile anaerobic microbes and binds heavy metals such as lead, mercury, and cadmium. It also exudes chlorinated hydrocarbons. These pesticides rank among the "dirty dozen" of the United Nations Environment Program. Spirulina contains about 1% chlorophyll.

Polysaccharides help to regulate the blood sugar level

Spirulina contains 15% of these high molecular carbohydrates, mainly in the form of rhamnose and the reserve-carb glycogen playing an important role in the regulation of blood sugar levels. Polysaccharides stimulate the cellular immunity by increasing the production of macrophages (large phagocytes) and the killer and helper cells.

In 1996 Hayashi and his colleagues found out that a water extract of the blue-green algae (calcium spirulan) inhibits the replication of HIV-I, herpes simplex, and other viruses. The antiviral effect could Hayashi confirm 2008 at the University of Toyama, Japan, even in the replication stage after penetration into the cells of the virus formation. Calcium spirulan keeps the membranes of the cells of the immune system flexible. Thus, the viruses are no longer able to dock with the cell walls and penetrate the cells. In 2009, Tunisian researchers around Majdaub discovered the anticoagulant factor of calcium spirulan.

In addition to the antiviral and antibacterial activity of Spirulina, polysaccharides affect the blood clotting. At the University of Kiel, Matthias Peschanel showed promising results on tests with tumor cells (1996).

In 2013 Kawanishi and his Japanese research colleagues could prove that the complex polysaccharides in Spirulina suppress dangerous brain tumors. Akira Tominaga and his Japanese colleagues of the Kochi University analyzed the damage of human epithelial cells and their reconstruction with Spirulina's complex polysaccharides. They used human quasi-normal FPCK-1-1-cells from a colon polyp in a patient with familial increased incidence of initially benign polyps. The researchers suggest that the complex polysaccharides in Spirulina may be useful in preventing intestinal damage (2013).

Gamma-linolenic acid inhibits inflammations and regulates hormones

Fatty acids are the components of which fats and oils are combined. The body needs fats but only those which it can not produce itself: namely essential fatty acids, vitamin F or EFA. The EFA abundant in Spirulina are precursors of prostaglandins. The latter hormone-like chemicals act as messengers and regulators in many different body processes. They make for beautiful skin and hair as well as for low blood pressure, cholesterol and triglyceride levels. The brain needs EFA for normal development and functioning. EFA also helps with cardiovascular diseases, candida, eczema, and psoriasis.

Spirulina contains more than 5% of lipids or fats, mainly essential fatty acids. In the analysis, on page 7, only the most important are listed, the linoleic and gamma-linolenic acid

(GLA). Together they make up 211 mg per tablespoon Spirulina powder. Other essential fatty acids present in the algae are DHA, GLA, and dihomo gamma-linolenic acid. Gupta and his Indian fellow researchers found in 2010 that the treatment with Spirulina reduces the risk of osteoporosis by the antidiabetic rosiglitazone.

Spirulina contains 110 mg gamma-linolenic acid, otherwise, only found in breast milk and oil extracts of evening primrose, hemp, borage seeds, and black currants. A 500 mg capsule of evening primrose oil contains 45 mg. GLA acid helps regulate the entire hormonal system.

Alcohol and animal fats excluding fish oil can cause a lack of GLA. Studies show that such a deficiency can lead to many health problems. Therefore a food source such as Spirulina is particularly important.

- Polysaccharides help with diabetes and cold sores; they also boost the immunity.
- Gamma-linolenic acid (GLA) regulates hormones, ensures good skin and circulation and fights candida.

Sulfolipids and glycolipids act against cancer and AIDS

40% of the lipids in Spirulina are glycolipids and about 2% sulfolipids, a proven valuable substance for people suffering from cancer or AIDS. In 1989, the National Cancer Institute (NCI) initiated a study. Kirk R. Gustafson and his research colleagues found out that the sulfonic parts of the glycolipids in Spirulina showed remarkably effective against the human immunodeficiency virus: They protect the T-cells against the toxic effect of HIV-1. Meanwhile, 27 years have passed and one should think many Spirulina studies with AIDS patients should have followed. Unfortunately, there were only a few. In 1989, Terry L. Pulse led one with 28 patients suffering from full blown AIDS. Apparently, he wanted to confirm Gustafson's test tube study in humans. 16 patients showed significant improvements: 2 were HIV-negative after 180 days, 5 followed later! Are these findings used in traditional medicine? Is Spirulina recognized as an immune booster? No way, Jose! Why are the billions in HIV/AIDS funding used primarily to bring even more chemical drugs on the market? Luckily, we can get info on the Internet of the causes of AIDS. Many rely on natural healers for boosting immunity. This disease is slowly serving its time as a love killer and scaremongering. So nothing seems to stand in the way of the procreation of future taxpayers except for decreasing sperm counts due to chemicals in the food and the environment and the fear of an uncertain future with low-paid jobs. In both matters, the detoxifying and exhilarating acting algae help. For job worries and progressive ways of working a machine or value-added tax and a basic citizen's income coupled with the replacement of the Labor and Employment Law could help. But only if it replaces all other transfer payments and the bureaucracies that oversee them. Then even the national debt might be cut.

Spirulina has been used as a dietary supplement in a recent study to improve the nutritional status of people living with HIV/AIDS. This study also confirms Spirulina's immunostimulating effect. In a three-month study in Giessen, Germany, Frank Winter and his team tested 73 women with an acquired immune deficiency. In the group receiving 5 g Spirulina daily the antioxidant capacity significantly improved (2014).

Let's not spend money on destructive drugs or we may finance our suffering and take part in possibly the largest mass extinction of all times. In Africa, it has already shown devastating effects. Or do we need the epidemics because of overpopulation? This at least suggested the chief oncologist at a university hospital after I had offered him a lot of the proven anti-cancer algae for his cancer- stricken young patients.

Spirulina's vitamins prevent deficiency diseases

In the human body, the vitamins work as active ingredients along with the enzymes providing adequate body functions. The human body rarely synthesizes vitamins. From the biochemical point of view, we should receive them regularly with the food. Natural nutrients from wild and medicinal herbs, trees and crops, Spirulina and other concentrated food supplements are preferable to synthetic multivitamins because artificial sweeteners are suspected to cause allergies and other side effects. Also, there may be overdoses in the fat-soluble vitamins A, D, E and K as these are stored mainly in the liver. Spirulina contains all these valuable nutrients in a balanced composition.

Pro-vitamin A (Carotinoids)	It prevents night blindness and eye diseases. Carotinoids reduce the risk of getting cancer.
Vitamin E (α-Tocopherol)	As "rust inhibitor" it protects fats from oxidizing and prevents age spots. Vitamin E improves oxygen analysis and a positive effect on blood count, fertility, muscles, and brain.
Vitamin B$_1$ (Thiamine)	Thiamine promotes the function of nerves and muscles including the heart muscle. A deficiency leads to beriberi, possibly caused by an extremely unbalanced diet or alcohol addiction. Symptoms include edema, enlargement of the liver, heavy breathing, numb hands, and feet, nervousness, and weakness.
Vitamin B$_2$ (Riboflavin)	It plays an essential role in the breakdown and utilization of carbohydrates, fats, and proteins. It provides energy, a healthy skin, and good eyes. The consumption of alcohol, birth control pills, and antidepressants may cause deficiencies such as brittle, dry lips, sore mouth, sensitivity to light and impaired vision.
Vitamin B$_3$ (Niacin)	Nicotinic acid and nicotinamide (vitamin B3) can be synthesized from the amino acid tryptophan. Niacin is involved in the functioning of the nervous and digestive system as well as in brain metabolism. It acts as a vasodilator and is essential for cellular respiration and energy. A deficiency can cause pellagra with the symptoms pustules, diarrhea, headache, and depression.
Vitamin B$_5$ (Pantothenic acid)	The "anti-stress vitamin" is involved in the production of anti-inflammatory and food utilizing corticosteroids and sex hormones. It strengthens the defense force and makes you fit and slim. Consuming precooked food, white flour, sugar, and alcohol may develop a vitamin B5 deficiency. Symptoms are fatigue, headache, nausea, tingling, numbness, abdominal pain, muscle spasms,

	and susceptibility to respiratory infections.
Vitamin B$_6$ (Pyridox-ine)	Pyridoxin is involved in protein and fat digestion. It promotes growth, provides good nerves, has a dehydrating effect and strengthens the immune system. An extremely high protein intake, excessive alcohol consumption, and physical exertion or taking birth control pills or pain-killers may lead to a deficiency. Symptoms are a sore mouth, frequent infections, irritability, melancholy, and poor skin.
Vitamin B$_{12}$ (Cobala-min)	Cobalamin is formed by microorganisms and as the only water-soluble vitamin stored in the body. Thus, the supply can be secured for many years if no massive gastric or intestinal damage are present. The latter could result in the lack of the intrinsic factor, a glycoprotein needed for vitamin B12 absorption. Cobalamin promotes the production of red blood cells in the bone marrow, provides for a functioning nervous system and is required for cell division and the activation of folic acid. Deficiency symptoms are skin / mucosal damage, nerve disorders, anemia, pallor, loss of appetite, intestinal damage diarrhea, irritability, fatigue.
Biotin (Vitamin H)	Biotin is essential for the skin, hair growth and central nervous system. It helps to relieve muscle pain. The cause of a deficiency is usually a damaged intestinal flora.
Inositol	Inositol acts against neurasthenia and anxiety. It helps in disorders of the liver metabolism, especially with fatty liver. It stimulates the gastrointestinal activity, prevents arteriosclerosis and is essential for sperm production.
Folic acid	It is essential for brain growth and reproduction. Folic acid prevents miscarriages and damage to the fetus. ensures the production of red blood cells and the functioning of the nervous system. A deficiency of this vitamin, combined with iron deficiency, is the most common vitamin deficiency in the Western industrialized countries. It is caused by alcohol and taking pills as well as by eating overcooked and fried food.

The alga's alkalizing and harmonizing minerals

Growing plants need the elements of dust that have formed over millions of years from abraded rock. We need plant minerals for a balanced composition of body fluids, to build bones and blood and to tone the muscles and cardiovascular system. As the vitamins, the minerals act as coenzymes. They are involved in all enzymatic activities and enable the body to perform its functions. Missing a single salt affects the ratio of the other salts. If this imbalance is not corrected, the subsequent chain reaction can lead to diseases. Spirulina contains a balanced selection of minerals and trace elements in a bioavailable form. Only minerals metabolized by plants are optimal assimilated by the organism. In contrast mineral salt supplements often cause deposits and inflammation. Next to Spirulina we can obtain the basic mood elevators from the green leafy plants, especially from weeds. Unfortunately, we live rarely close to zero-emission meadows to ensure daily supplies. Therefore we are very fortunate that Spirulina provides us with the following minerals without exhaust fumes and pesticides:

Boron	Boron is not included in the analysis but like other not listed elements also available in Spirulina. It helps to build muscles, provides for good brain functions, promotes calcium uptake and thus prevents osteoporosis after menopause.
Calcium	It forms solid bones and teeth, ensures regular heartbeat and transmission of nerve impulses. It lowers cholesterol and helps prevent cancer, osteoporosis and cardiovascular disease before. C. activates various enzymes and is involved in the RNA-DNA structure.
Chromium	It protects against diseases of the coronary arteries, provides energy, balances blood sugar fluctuations and prevents arteriosclerosis. Chromium promotes the breakdown of fat and muscle tissue. It can help against osteoporosis and contribute to the prolongation of life.
Iron	Iron carries oxygen to the cells and provides for the removal of carbon dioxide to the lungs. It is essential for the formation of the red blood pigment hemoglobin and the muscle pigment myoglobin. The hematopoietic salt prevents anemia and boosts the immune system.
Germanium	It is essential for the brain and helps to fight degenerative diseases. It derives cadmium and mercury, promotes the oxygenation of the tissues and prevents strokes. Also, germanium improves arthritis, cancer, candida, chronic viral infections, and AIDS.
Potassium	Potassium promotes healthy nerves and regulates the water balance, blood pressure, and heartbeat. It helps to prevent strokes and to promote adequate muscle contractions. Diuretics, diarrhea, vomit, and laxatives can cause potassium loss.
Copper	It is an essential component of many enzymes. Copper helps to build bones, red blood cells, and hemoglobin. Together with zinc and vitamin C, it forms elastin. It helps against osteoporosis, is involved in the pigmentation of the skin and hair as well as in the sensation of

	taste. It promotes healthy nerves and joints.
Lithium	Lithium is one of the psychotropic drugs and used for the prevention and treatment of manic-depressive conditions.
Magnesium	It forms bones and teeth and ensures adequate muscle contraction. It is essential for the transmission of nerve impulses and the activation of energy-producing enzymes. It helps to keep the pH in the normal range and to prevent cardiovascular diseases, osteoporosis, and some cancers. The basic salt lifts the spirits and stables the nerves.
Manganese	We need Manganese for protein and fat metabolism, a healthy immune system, and for healthy nerves; as well as for energy production, the growth of the bone and the reproduction. M. helps to build cartilage and synovia.
Molybdenum	Molybdenum provides in minimum doses for nitrogen metabolism and helps in the latter stages of the conversion of purines to uric acid. A deficiency can lead to cancer or mouth and palate complaints.
Selenium	Together with Vitamin E, Selenium keeps the heart and liver healthy. As a powerful antioxidant, it prevents the oxidation of fats and the formation of free radicals. S. prevents some types of tumors. It ensures a functioning pancreas and the elasticity of the tissue.
Zinc	Zinc ensures the protein synthesis, the collagen structure, and a healthy immune system. It promotes wound healing as well as the sense of smell and taste. Zinc is essential for the reproductive organs and prevents arteriosclerosis and cancer.

Spirulina's unique profile of amino acids

Air and water are polluted. The soil is used and poisoned, lacking trace elements. More than a quarter century ago, tests already revealed a dangerous low amino acid (AA) profile in the body (Bragg and Bragg 1992). To protect ourselves from this deficiency, we better consume the controlled organic food and pollution-free, protein-rich microalgae as a food supplement. Missing a single AA the body can not properly carry out protein synthesis possibly leading to growth and digestion disorders or depression. Such disorders may also occur in a balanced diet containing enough protein since the lack of available essential AA can also be caused by chemical drugs, infections, impaired absorption or by traumatic events. In this case, you can benefit from Spirulina's detoxifying, anti-inflammatory, digestive, and mood-lifting effect. It contains all the essential AA in the exact composition of the human body and its needs. These are responsible for protein structure, blood formation, growth, healing and repair of muscle tissue, structure of the bone, the collagen, and connective tissue, stabilizing the blood sugar and energy level as well as the hormonal balance, strengthen the nervous system and the immune system.

To include all functions, I'd have to add many pages because amino acids are the building blocks from which all proteins are constructed, providing the structure of all living things and taking part in all vital processes.

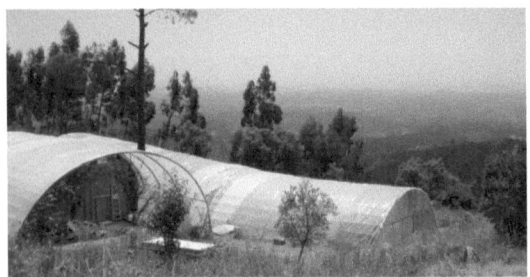

https://www.workaway.info/595215223583-en.html

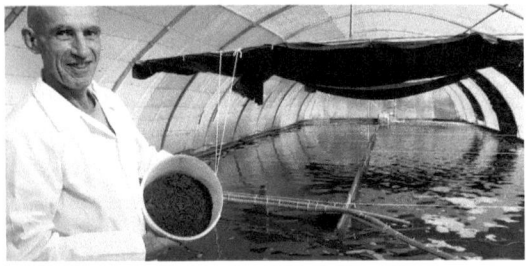

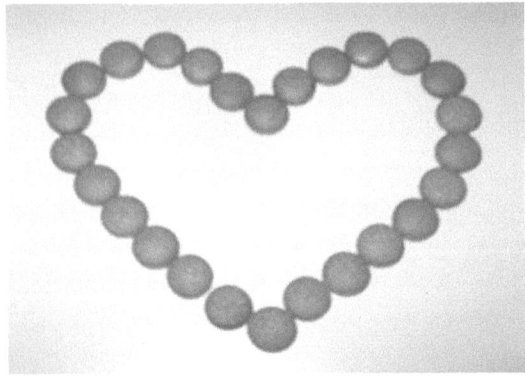

V. SPIRULINA'S HEALTH-PROMOTING EFFECTS

Why do we live longer than our ancestors?

Before presenting the algae as a natural healer, I respond to a question I am frequently asked: If environmental toxins and food are ever so bad for us, why do we live longer than at times when the food was still natural? In fact, the life expectancy is higher than 100 years ago. But at what price? Look at nursing homes and judge for yourself whether the elderly live there or waste away slowly and painfully. The question why we are living longer can be answered by statistics: Chinese and Americans have about the same life expectancy however with a serious difference: The US Americans have from the 50th year a significantly higher risk of developing allergies, Alzheimer's, cardiovascular failure, cancer, Parkinson's, rheumatism and other modern plagues. As the difference between the two nations, the statistics have discovered the storage of foodstuffs and food chemistry. While Americans have long existed of preserved food, the Chinese lived until recently exclusively from fresh or naturally preserved foods meaning: Preservatives make not only the food but also their consumers durable. Since artificial sweeteners are due to their too large molecules less well absorbed by the cells as natural ones, they accumulate in the body resulting in health problems. This sad truth answers the question why the western elderly live longer wasting away.

Now how can the spiral microorganism help us? An increasingly dense network of scientific studies confirms its effect diversity. On universities and other research centers around the world, the blue-green algae are studied for their therapeutic effects with more than promising results.

Before you use Spirulina in a case of illness, an intestinal cleansing is highly recommended. Only then are the valuable nutrients of the microorganism completely absorbed. Otherwise, they are only producing precious excrement and expensive urine. Diseases base on slagged intestinal walls. These incrustations have to be loosened first.

How you can do it, you find on p. 27, chapter Colon and liver cleansing.

Spirulina strengthens your immune system

A revealing study in humans has confirmed Spirulina's immunostimulatory effect. Frank Winter and his team tested in the three-month Gießen study 73 women with acquired immune deficiency. In the group given 5 g Spirulina daily, the antioxidant capacity was significantly improved (2014).

Also, Marthe-Elise Ngo-Matip and her 7-member team confirmed the alga's immune-boosting effect. They conducted a 12-month study with 320 HIV-1-infected individuals in the former German colony of Cameroon. In the group receiving Spirulina, the CD4 cells increased after 6 months significantly, and the viral load decreased noticeably. After one year, the hemoglobin levels were significantly higher in the Spirulina group, while the fasting blood glucose concentration was significantly lower compared to the control group (2015). Other countless studies around the globe revealed: The natural orange-red, blue and green pigments of Spirulina, beta-carotene, phycocyanin, and chlorophyll stimulate the immune system and the cell control or cell communication. They selectively destroy cancer cells and act as antioxidants. In 1998, Mishima and colleagues showed that a sulfated polysaccharide of Spirulina (calcium spirulan) inhibits the invasion and metastasis of tumors.

Other immunostimulatory components are iron, germanium, manganese, zinc and numerous enzymes. They inhibit inflammation and trigger immune complexes. Vitamin B6 (pyridoxine) also helps with immune functions and antibody production. The high content of the antioxidant vitamin E, the anti-inflammatory gamma-linolenic acid and the amino acids lysine, methionine, and threonine increase and activate the immune cells so strengthen the immune system. In 1987, Japanese researchers found out: 5% Spirulina in the diet of animals increased the lactobacilli in an intestinal section three times more than in the control group. The beneficial microorganisms in the intestinal flora render invading germs harmless. Chemical drugs destroy those friendly bacteria belonging to the natural defense of our body. Therefore you better consume Spirulina if you take chemical drugs such as painkillers or the pill.

Danish researchers working with Morten Lobner give an example of a study without torturing the creature: They identified 11 men with an altered response of white blood cells to two antigens: Candida albicans and tetanus toxoid. Spirulina caused a strong temporary immune response apparently by generating a pre-inflammatory stage (2008).

Recently, Cuban researchers confirmed an immune response in rats against cell damage induced by H_2O_2 and glutamate. Javier Marin-Prida and his team found: Spirulina's phycocyanin promotes cell survival. It corrects immune and inflammatory genes and oxidative stress markers in acute hypoperfusion of rat brains. These results suggest that phycocyanin has the potential to treat ischemic, so by hypoperfusion caused strokes (2013).

- Spirulina propagates and activates white blood cells and destroys cancer cells.
- SOD and other enzymes act as strong antioxidants inhibiting inflammation and dissolve immune complexes.
- The alga builds up a beneficial intestinal flora and strengthens the immune system.

The alga helps with hypertension, obesity, and diabetes

Japanese researchers confirmed the algae's blood pressure lowering effect (Iwata et al. 1990). Also, a new study by Lu and colleagues at the Tokyo University shows: Spirulina is suitable for preventing and treating high blood pressure (2010). Ichimura and his team from the University of Nagasaki confirmed an anti-hypertensive effect of Spirulina's blue pigment (2013). Regrettably, these findings are ignored by conventional medicine.

Participants of my questionnaire study and several Spirulina consumers confirm this effect. See also *SPIRULINA EXPERIENCES AROUND THE GLOBE*, pages 71 et seqq.

Diabetics are supposed to eat more vegetable protein but less fat and calories. Spirulina contains 60 - 65 % easily digestible protein, less than 6 % fat and no calories. Especially valuable for people with out-of-control blood sugar are Spirulina's polysaccharides stored in the body as glycogen and converted into glucose if needed or turned back to glycogen. If too much glucose (sugar) is in the blood, the excess is converted into glycogen and stored in the liver and muscles. If the blood sugar is too low, glycogen is converted back to glucose and released into the blood.

Spirulina also contains the amino acid leucine and organically bound, therefore, well absorbable chromium. As a coenzyme, chromium activates insulin. It relieves the pancreas and balances blood sugar fluctuations. In inorganic form, e. g., as chromium tablets, the trace element is less well absorbed by the body. Spirulina's extremely high proportion of the neurotransmitter glutamic acid also helps that it does not come to a lowering of blood sugar in the complex treatment of diabetes.

Since the alga inhibits the craving for white flour and sugar it is apt for diabetics in two respects: Empty calories from sweet paste foods, mostly heated starch, reduce chromium levels leading to overloading the pancreas as it must produce large amounts of insulin.

Japanese researchers concluded: A water-soluble part of Spirulina lowers blood sugar levels, while the water-insoluble part keeps it low when loaded with sugar (Takai et al. 1991). Chinese researchers found that the polysaccharides in Spirulina can reduce the blood glucose level and protect the blood vessels (Huang et al. 2005). In recent years, scientists from China, India, Brazil, Egypt, and other countries have confirmed the glucose-lowering effect of various components in Spirulina. In 2013, researchers at the Pharmaceutical University in Nanjing, China, discovered the anti-diabetic potential of Spirulina's phycocyanin in diabetes-2. (Ou et al.)

In 1986, E. W. Becker and his colleagues demonstrated the appetite-reducing effect of the algae. The male subjects of the study received 2.8 g Spirulina 3 times a day as a dietary supplement for four weeks. They could significantly reduce their weight compared to the control group who received a placebo. In 2010, Maria Kalafati and her colleagues published their Spirulina study in the journal Medicine & Science. They tested the endurance of people. In only 4 weeks the researchers found a significant improvement in performance in the men who received a dose of 6 g Spirulina per day. At that, the exercise performance increased probably due to the increased fat burning and the increased level of the radical scavenger glutathione.

• Spirulina's polysaccharides, chromium, glutamic acid and the amino acid leucine ensure a balanced blood sugar level.

• In 1986, the appetite-reducing effect of the algae was found.

• 1990, 2010, and 2013 scientists demonstrated the blood pressure lowering effect of the cyanobacteria.

Spirulina detoxes and protects the nerves

Toxins can cause numerous so-called civilization diseases such as MS, Parkinson's, AIDS, Alzheimer's disease, eczema or shingles, regardless of whether taken in for a long period of time in small doses or at once. Artificial sweeteners overburden the immune system, lead to chronic fatigue, inefficiency or nerve damages. Researchers at the Faculty of Pharmacy of the University of Madrid view Spirulina as a useful tool for the development of a new treatment of neurodegenerative disorders such as Alzheimer's or Parkinson (Bermejo-Bescos et al. 2008).

Spirulina's emunctory effect of heavy metals, metabolic poisons and chemicals have been repeatedly scientifically proven by Fukino and other researchers. See chapter Detox with Spirulina. If you work with pesticides or eat few organic vegetables, you better take Spirulina and drink plenty of pure water even if Parkinson, MS or other modern diseases have developed. The acidification of the body fluids causes the acid crystals to abrade the delicate nerve endings and cause inflammation of the nerves. Result: The neural function is limited, and the transmission of impulses from the brain to the muscles interrupted.

Indian researchers found out that Spirulina reduces fluoride poisoning (Banji 2013). See chapter The blue-green light carrier cures AIDS.

The Vitamin B6 in Spirulina (pyridoxine) supports the nervous system, and B12 (cobalamin) builds the protective coating of the nerve cells. The glycolipids are also useful for the myelin sheaths of the nervous tissue. They are the very components of the cell membrane that form membrane receptors mainly in the myelin sheath of the nerve tissue. Those receiving and transferring facilities control various physiological and biochemical processes. Spirulina's minerals calcium and magnesium reduce stress acids, help against depression and provide for good nerves. See chapter Spirulina - soul balm for the new age.

• Toxins in the body can cause MS, Parkinson, Alzheimer and other diseases.

• Spirulina helps to eliminate toxic salts and heavy metals.

• The alga builds a protective layer of the nerve cells.

• The basic fare prevents acidosis and nerve damage.

Prompt help for allergic reactions

Allergies indicate that the body is poisoned and slagged already up to the brim. Chemical drugs which inhibit the production of histamine (antihistamines) would strain the body additionally. Therefore, it makes sense to use the antiallergic acting spiral algae regularly.

From my experience, I know how quickly Spirulina provides relief with hypersensitivity reactions. Without the natural healer, I would suffer from severe hay fever, food chemistry, and pet hair allergy. If I forget a few days to eat Spirulina, my eyes itch when petting cats, and much more being near rabbits. Sometimes I feel like choking on mucus when I eat certain convenience foods. Sucking 3 to 4 Spirulina tabs or drinking fruit juice with some algae powder, I'm free of symptoms after two to three minutes. Spirulina and pure water bring people with asthma and allergy rapid relief.

If you drink non-carbonated H2O, the cells throttle the histamine production. Components of Spirulina also inhibit the emission of the mast cell granules of the skin tissue which contain histamine reducing the skin's reactivity. Spirulina gets to the root of all evil by detoxifying the body.

Around the globe, researchers tested the algae's anti-allergic effect. In 2001, German scientists discovered a combination of the trace element zinc and the amino acid histidine can stop hay fever. Prof. Rudolf Schopf accounts a lack of zinc jointly responsible since it has direct anti-allergic properties. Spirulina contains zinc, histidine and a number of other substances acting against allergies. In 1997, the South Korean researchers Yang, Lee, and Kim presented the beneficial mite may even act lifesaving since it completely suppresses the anaphylactic shock at a dose of ½ to 1 mg per kilogram body weight. This allergic reaction to penicillin or wasp stings belongs to the

immediate reaction of the allergy type I, as well as hay fever, animal hair allergy, asthma, and hives.

In 1998, Kim and his team proved Spirulina's inhibitory effect of mast cell mediated allergic reactions of the immediate type.

In 2005, Californian researchers led by Mao demonstrated the benefits of Spirulina in patients with allergic rhinitis.

In 2008, Cemal Cingi and his Turkish fellow researchers could determine efficacy in allergic rhinitis in a double-blind, placebo-controlled study. The symptoms such as nasal discharge, sneezing, nasal congestion, and itching improved in the Spirulina group significantly compared to placebo.

- Allergies are caused by poisons and slagging.
- Spirulina relieves hay fever symptoms such as nasal discharge, sneezing, and itching.
- ½ -1 g Spirulina per kg body weight suppresses the anaphylactic shock to 100%.

The blue-green light carrier cures AIDS

We can all get AIDS not only heroin addicts and homosexuals. As the name, Acquired Immuno Deficiency Syndrome suggests it is a nonheritable immunological disorder with reduced resistance to infectious disease. It takes years to destroy the immune system if you do not supply the body with the necessary nutrients or use unnatural substances. In 1982, the Morbidity and Mortality Weekly Report showed: In the first US cities where the tab water was fluoridated, in New York, San Francisco, and Miami, four times more cases of AIDS appeared than in the still not fluoridated cities Newark, Houston, and Los Angeles.

David Banji and his Indian colleagues from the Department of Pharmacology and Toxicology in Nalgonda found that supplementation with Spirulina during pregnancy reduced the toxicity risk of fluoride in the offspring of rats (2013). If we supply the body with fluoridated water, salt, and toothpaste we are well advised to consume Spirulina for detoxification regularly.

Alternative physicians such as Dr. Matthias Rath and many microbiologists and vaccination critics view the cause of AIDS as a vitamin deficiency. Some time ago, we saw on TV a man in a Frankfurt shelter for AIDS patients. He like every day fried a pan full of steaks, and neither ate vegetables nor salad with it and was surprised that he got no power of all the dead meat! By contrast, the funny Dr. Eckart von Hirschhausen is surprised about the fact that there are still no suppositories of the only immune-enhancing animal food, the chicken soup. That too much red meat is robbing us our juice and power rickshaw drivers have learned. With meat consumption, it was difficult for them to pedal.

Also, if we daily consume illegal or legal drugs or chemical medicines, we lose vitamins and in the long run the body's defense. Likewise, promiscuous behavior leads to immunodeficiency because the immune system is overloaded with foreign protein.

If we treat the consequential infections with chemical mace in the form of antibiotics, antifungal agents, and steroids we weaken the body's defense further. Also, the anal intercourse constantly strains the immune system since the skin of the anus is unlike the padded vagina thin and tears easily. The immune system constantly works in extra shifts to repair these injuries. Over the years the defenses get steadily weaker also due to anal penetration-facilitating drugs. The Stuttgart molecular biologist Dr. Stefan Lanka suspects:

Nitrites (poppers) and common AIDS drugs are destroying the immune system in the long run. This is also evident by the fact that long-term survivors tested HIV-positive for 10-20 years without getting AIDS. They refuse to nearly 100% chemical drugs by taking alternative medicine. Studies in Frankfurt, Chicago, Boston, and London testify to positive results of such remedies (Zur Lippe and Hauber et al. 1997).

Epidemiological evidence points to the connection between poppers and the development of AIDS. In particular, they cause Kaposi's sarcoma. Poppers or nitrites (amyl or isobutyl) destroy the immune system reducing the blood's ability to carry oxygen thus causing anemia. They are used to increase the blood flow to the penis and the threshold of pain and relax the smooth anal muscles. Poppers also increase the feeling of orgasm and trigger mild intoxication in the brain. Poppers are primarily but not exclusively used by homosexuals. I recommend reading the science-based book by Dr. med. Heinrich Kremer "The Silent Revolution in Cancer and AIDS medicine". Kremer urgently warns against the official "AIDS treatments" as they come up to "an Acquired Iatrogenic Death Syndrome (AIDS), so an acquired Death Syndrome forced by doctors".

For seven years, I voluntarily gave Reiki in the AIDS support group founded by Louise Hay and wanted to verify the in vitro study conducted by Gustafson on the 250-300 mostly young men who every Wednesday met on San Vincente Boulevard in West Hollywood. However, since too few long-term survivors provided information, I forwarded the questionnaires to individuals with immunodeficiency and immune deficiency diseases. Halima Neumann (see also page 98) handed on around 30 questionnaires to patients who completed her deacidification seminars. Besides Spirulina, you can use echinacea, hypericin (main active ingredient hypericum, concentrated in Jarsin300), glycyrrhiza (licorice), viola, and ginkgo to rebuild the immune system.

The long-term survivors of my study also reject chemical drugs. They pay attention to healthy eating and physical activity. They also have steady jobs.

Spirulina is an ideal food and cure for AIDS patients. The alga builds up the immune system systematically and provides the body with much-needed nutrients and more than 60 % cell-regenerating protein of the highest quality without burdening the organism by heavy work of digestion. And since Spirulina

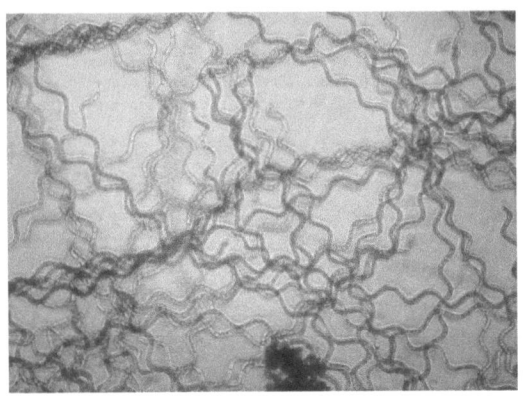

lifts the mood, it is a blessing for all people suffering from any health condition.

Studies around the globe proof: The regular consumption of Spirulina causes the so-called "HIV" positives to test negative.

I use apostrophes because I doubt that HIV exists at all or causes AIDS. Several microbiologists assert that so far no scientists have succeeded in isolating the so-called HIV (Human Immunodeficiency Virus). The HIV photos contain no genetically analyzed only virus-like particles.

Nevertheless, the disease industry further fans the fear of contagion on false assumptions. Unprotected love-making is criminalized. The predictions of the epidemics gurus have after 30 years not come to hand. GRID, the disease mainly occurring among drug addicts and homosexuals (Gay Related Immune Deficiency) would exterminate vast sections of the population as in medieval times should no suitable medication and vaccines are being developed.

Though of course, the disease industry has not come up with a vaccine against body-misuse the inhabitants of Europe remained about the same. It seems AIDS research is degenerating in a workshop for muddle-heads. No wonder the specialists all disagree: There is no scientific logic behind the AIDS tales. Why?

The standard HIV test procedures according to the manufacturer are unreliable. If you suffer from severe rheumatoid arthritis, MS in the late stage, skin-TBC, cancer, lupus, herpes or severe chronic alcoholism you can test positive. Tests are anyway only positive for the disease industry. For patients, they are mainly stirring up fear which blocks as the largest stressor additionally immune functions and consume a lot of energy.

On the other hand, viruses are not responsible for chronic diseases. The alleged human immunodeficiency virus can't be contagious otherwise men and women would be equally affected. But only in Africa, the continent of the banned pesticides, vitamin deficiencies, mutilations, potheads, and drug users AIDS is not spread gender specific. Why over here the ratio of male and female AIDS patients altered since the 1980s from 90:10 to 80:20 is partly due to the rise in cosmetic surgery, tattoos, piercing, anal sex and other the immune system debilitating sexual practices.

Since fantasies are hardly ever been photographed, there is no pic of the phantom virus only cell debris or cell particles sold as HIV photos. You will suffer from immunodeficiency when you abuse your body with drugs or alcohol, worry excessively and constantly submit to bloody beauty manipulations or other fashion or macho dictations.

The biggest problem for people suffering from AIDS is the lack of appetite and the associated risk not to supply the body with the sufficient quantity of protein needed for the build-up of the endogenous protein.

In that respect, Spirulina serves you best. 3 times daily ¼ liter fruit or vegetable juice or broth with 1 tbsp of Spirulina powder regenerates your immune system, takes care of your mental and spiritual well-being, relieves anxiety and harmonizes the organism.

So better trust your inner healer rather than to acidify your body with chemicals. If you drink pure water, eat living food, soak up the sun's energy, move in the fresh air and do not forget mental activity and rest you live according to the laws of nature. Then the self-regulation of the organism sets in again since our inner healer quests for homeostasis, keeping a constant inner milieu.

- In the first US cities where tap water was fluoridated AIDS occurred four times more than in non-fluoridated cities.
- With drug abuse and lack of nutrients and vitamins, you destroy the immune system in about 10-15 years.
- Medicinal director em. Dr. Kremer calls AIDS a forced physicians death syndrome.
- Promiscuous behavior overtaxes the immune system with a permanent input of foreign protein.
- HIV tests are questionable due to high false-positive-rates.
- Anal sex constantly ruptures the thin skin of the rectum weakening the body's defense. The same applies for repeated lifting, wrinkle-injections, piercing, and tattooing.
- With regular Spirulina consumption so-called HIV-positives test in time HIV-negative having a 0 quota on the MWR-scale.

Spirulina heals wounds and acts as antibiotic

As early as the 60s and 70s, researchers from around the world were able to demonstrate the following: Spirulina accelerates wound healing, promotes skin metabolism, reduces scarring and inhibits the growth of bacteria, yeasts and fungi (Clement 1967, Martinez Nadal 1970, Yoshida 1977 Jorjani and Amirani 1978). Also, Spirulina increasingly produces antibodies (Hayashi 1998) and prevents replication of several enveloped viruses such as herpes simplex 1 (cause of cold sores), HCV (human cytomegalovirus), measles and mumps, the HIV (Hayashi et al. 1994 and 1996) and the influenza virus type A from which worldwide arise new strains due to instability. The type A virus triggers the most severe form of influenza. Having the flu more than once a year or suffering from reoccurring cold sores indicates an immunodeficiency. In this case, it would be best to use the blue-green light food regularly as it evidently strengthens the immune system.

At the first tingling and burning dab the lips immediately with an aqueous Spirulina solution

or with a humidified Spirulina tablet. In addition, it is essential to eat lysine-rich foods such as avocados, beans, buckwheat, organic eggs and cream cheese and to avoid arginine-containing foods, especially nuts, and chocolate. We can also take higher doses of the amino acid lysine to prevent a herpes outbreak. A few years ago I created recipes for my book on cranberry with the bladder protecting berry. Taking cranberry capsules as an additional immune booster protects against cold sores and cystitis. Also, 65% (53 people) of the participants of my ongoing study of currently 84 volunteers indicated with Spirulina to have improved immune function or less frequently suffer from infections.

- Spirulina inhibits the spread of viruses, bacteria, yeasts, and fungi.

- The algae force wound healing and reduce scarring.
- Spirulina improves the immune function.
- The microorganism helps with herpes simplex.

The micro-organism acts promptly against anemia

Pallor, fatigue, and shortness of breath indicate anemia. Menstruating and pregnant women, the elderly and malnourished as well as people suffering from peptic bleeding ulcers are often anemic. The most commonly occurring form of anemia is an iron deficiency anemia. Also, the lack of vitamin B12, folic acid, and vitamin E can lead to anemia. Studies in humans and animals prove Spirulina to be an excellent dietary supplement to correct this deficiency within a short time. It contains all above-mentioned nutrients including iron in the best bioavailable form essential for red blood cell formation.

Ms. Ursel C. from Lübeck send me an email on July 8. 2014:

"The blood analysis was sensational. I've never had such high levels of iron. Thanks, Spirulina!"

The absorption of the alga is in comparison to the conventional iron preparations by 60% higher (Takemoto 1982). Also, a single overdose of an over the counter drug can lead to death. (Galmén and Hojer (2014). The Swedish researchers reported that a 20-year old woman who was hospitalized 4 hours after absorbing iron, could not be saved.

Carlo Selmi and his team from the University of Davis in California and the Faculty of Medicine of the IRCCS in Milan Italy confirmed T. Takeuchi's study from 1978 with 8 young anemic women whose hemoglobin levels were normal after four weeks with 4 g Spirulina after each meal. This time 40 volunteers were tested 50 years and older. During the 12-week study period, the persons of both sexes had a steady increase in average hemoglobin levels (2011).

My study with patients suffering from immune deficiency showed that the subjects taking penicillin, sulfonamides, and cortisone had significant immune deficiencies and suffered from anemia. The anemic participants improved their blood levels after consuming Spirulina. They had normal hemoglobin levels. Given these findings, good doctors and healers suggest the algae as a hematopoietic cell regenerating supplementary food.

- The organically bound iron in Spirulina is better absorbed by the body than ordinary iron preparations.
- 4 g Spirulina after each meal fixes anemia in one month.
- Penicillin, sulfonamides, and cortisone lead to anemia.

Arthritis: with the blue-green algae rapidly free of complaints

The conventional medicine uses liver damage causing analgesics for the treatments of rheumatoid arthritis. Also, ibuprofen can cause gastrointestinal problems with bleeding and perforations. The side effects of the anti-inflammatory sulfonamide sulfapyridine used in treating painful joint inflammations are nausea, vomiting, loss of appetite and decreased absorption of the vitamin folic acid. In this respect, the natural supplement Spirulina guarantees the best results, shown by Mohamed M. Abdel-Daim and his Egyptian team even with colitis (2015). And yet are the side effects downright positive: energy boost, steady bowel movements, good liver counts, low blood sugar, blood pressure, and cholesterol, good mood and sleep, fewer calluses and age spots, moist, soft and elastic skin. I could go on filling pages. Also, Gabriel Gutierrez Rebolledo and his Mexican colleagues could, as many researchers before them, confirm the protective effect of the algae in chronic inflammation (2015).

Hundreds of millions of people suffer from prolonged or recurrent pain. About a quarter of them is highly suicidal because nothing can help. WHO has estimated that as many as 1 in 10 adults are newly diagnosed with chronic pain each year.
http://bmcpublichealth.biomedcentral.com/articles/10.1186/1471-2458-11-770

Spirulina is especially effective with joint pains usually caused by sweet, fat, and white paste food coupled with a lack of raw food, pure water, and exercise. Many researchers have confirmed the alga's anti-inflammatory effect. The participants of my ongoing study indicate to have fewer or even no more pain. 3 x 2 Spirulina tabs per day are enough to relieve or dissolve the pain. The anti-inflammatory substances are primarily the gamma-linolenic acid and the enzyme SOD. See page 39 et seqq.

Kirlian photographs, taken according to Peter Mandel before and after taking Spirulina, confirm the effect against inflammation. Many inflammation spots the doctor, and Naturopath Jürgen Görke had shown me on the first shot of my fingers and toes had disappeared on the 2nd though it was taken only 7 minutes after ingesting 7 algae tablets.

Researchers at the University Tempe, Arizona, USA, found in a pilot clinical trial that organic sulfur (methylsulfonylmethane - MSM; see also page 26 et seq.) gives the cartilage new strength. The sulfur content in Spirulina could, therefore, be the reason why the consumers of the microalgae improve their mobility and reduce their joint pain! (Kim 2006)

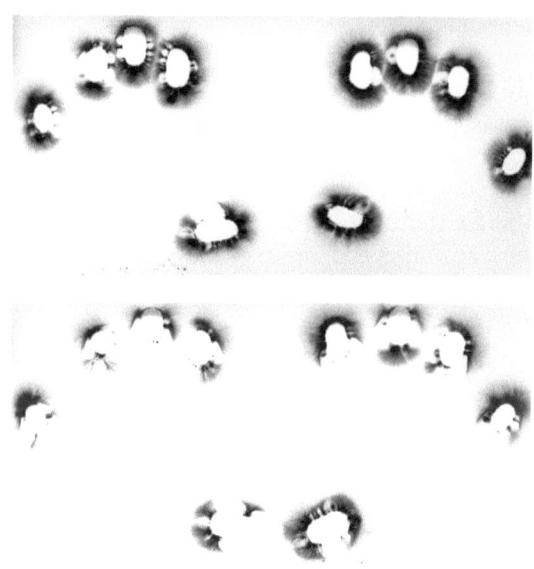

The alga protects from eye diseases

The retina of the eye needs vitamin A in the highest concentration. A deficiency manifests as night blindness, dry eyes, and frequent infections.

Excessive television and computer work can increase the need for vitamin A by a multiple. Spirulina contains umpteen times more carotenoids than carrots. In the intestinal walls, they are converted to vitamin A. These orange-red pigments protect the cells from the damaging effect of light such as UV rays. They also help with retinal sensitivity and night blindness. Spirulina is thus a valuable food for all people with eye problems.

A clinical report by Dr. Yoshito Yamazaki, a professor at the Tokyo College of Medicine and Dentistry demonstrated Spirulina improves vision in cataract, glaucoma, and retinal hemorrhage. This study with 480 participants proved the alga in 90 % of geriatric cataracts to be effective (Hills 1980). Rasiah Pratheepa Kumari and his Indian team could confirm Spirulina's retarding effect of cataract in vitro (in a test tube) and in vivo (in a living organism) (2013). Chinese ophthalmologists around L. Yang studied Spirulina's effect in vascularisation of the cornea. They pointed out the benefits of the algae in the treatment of diseases of the cornea and eye inflammation (2009).

In a study in India, 5000 preschool children received a daily dose of 1g Spirulina for 5 months. This amount is sufficient to meet the daily requirement of beta-carotene (provitamin A) or prevent blindness. The matt white Bitot's spots in the palpebral fissure of the conjunctiva decreased from 80% to 10% (Seshadri 1993).

Personal experience: Since the daily consumption of Spirulina I am free from conjunctivitis which I had often suffered due to drafts (open car window). My husband, an ex-racer and test driver, regularly takes Spirulina. When the old "Striezel" Stuck gained with his team in the early 21st century the 3rd place, he said that this was his most difficult 24-hour race. My hubby 9 years his senior raced five night hours through the *Green Hell*. Peters young co-racers were less fast in the dark, so he took some of their rounds with his Spirulina tuned eyes. Even better seems to be Astaxanthin. In 2012/13 I tested 8 bottles of the *king of carotenoids*. My eyes improved by 1 ½ & 4 diopters.

- With increased PC or TV use you need more vitamin A. The alga prevents conjunctivitis, cataract, glaucoma, and retinal bleeding.
- Spirulina's highly concentrated beta-carotene (Provitamin A) protects cells from damaging exposure to light (UV rays).

Spirulina prevents acidosis and hair loss

If we overload our humor with acids, we forfeit our hair and inner harmony. With regular consumption of the microalgae, cultured in soda water in a pH range from 8.5 to 11, we can prevent much suffering. Spirulina ensures a balanced acid-alkaline ratio.

Symptoms of body acidity

Insomnia, migraine, rheumatoid arthritis, frequent sighing, foul-smelling stool, sometimes hard and dry, sometimes as diarrhea, burning in the anus, decreased urination, tooth sensitivity when consuming acidic fruit or vinegar, burning in the mouth or under the tongue and hair loss. Hair loss is also associated with stress. In certain stages of life, when we are under physical and mental strain, hairs sometimes go out in clumps. In such situations, the basic algae help reduce the stress-based acid production.

Progress report: In early 1999, Rita S. complained about hair loss. For no apparent reason, her long hair began to go out and would no longer grow back. She had only about half of her hair left when she began to take Spirulina. After a few days, new hair sprouted. Two months later, they had a length of 2 to 3 cm.

- Our food and drinking water has an acid surplus which leads to blood acidity and loss of hair.
- Spirulina ensures an acid-alkaline balance, reduces stress-induces acids and promotes hair regrowth.

Spirulina helps to lower cholesterol

Several studies have shown: The blood of patients suffering from arteriosclerosis lack the lipolytic lipase and other enzymes. It is the reason for the cholesterol-lowering effect of the enzyme-rich algae. This demonstrated

Devi and Venkataraman and Kato et al. 1983 and 1984. Two years later, E. W. Becker and his team tested Spirulina's weight-reducing potential. The scientists of the University of Tübingen discovered the cholesterol lowering effect of the cyanobacterium by accident. In 1988, Nakaya and colleagues tested the algae at the Department of Internal Medicine at the University of Tokai on 30 male volunteers. With 4.2 g Spirulina per day the LDL cholesterol decreased in eight weeks from 243 mg/dl on average to 232.7 mg/dl. These results indicate that the regular consumption of Spirulina can reduce the risk of developing arteriosclerosis. Zbynek Strasky and his team from the Faculty of Pharmacy of the University of Prague also shared this positive prognosis end of 2013.

Low-density lipoproteins (LDL) are considered risk factors. High-density lipoproteins (HDL) protect against arterial diseases. The higher the HDL-count to the total cholesterol the better the ratio, e. g., total cholesterol 210 HDL 80 = 2.6. Although, the cholesterol is slightly increased but harmless due to the good ratio.

- The microorganism lowers cholesterol and prevents a heart attack.
- Spirulina lowers the bad cholesterol (LDL), thus reducing the risk of developing deposits in the arteries.

The Cyanobacteria has an antidepressant-like effect

It is known optimists live longer. In 2000, Toshihiko Maruta and his team found this out in a 30-year study at the Mayo Clinic. A lack of certain nutrients often leads to depression. Tablets for high blood pressure, antacids, water pills, painkillers, some heart medicine, antibiotics, and birth control pills can make indirect depressive or cause nutrients, such as vitamin C, vitamin B6 and B12, folic acid, magnesium, calcium or zinc to deplete. There is also evidence that depression and neurological problems are due to a deficiency of the amino acids phenylalanine, tyrosine, tryptophan or histidine. Phenylalanine increases the production of endorphins in the brain, thus helping to relieve stress and anxiety. Also, gastric congestion and lack of exercise can also lead to the blues. This doomsday scenario may evolve to melancholy. In his remarkable book, *Sugar Blues,* William Dufty made aware of the relationship between the addictive substance sugar and the susceptibility to diseases of all kinds, including depression, lack of concentration, and mental illness.

The alga is effective against depression. It cheers up, inhibits the craving for sweets, and less medication is needed.

Spirulina's excellent amino acid profile, the acid-buffering alkaline minerals and concentrated B- (stress) vitamins lift the spirits. They lead to harmony and wellbeing. The minerals calcium and magnesium activate the neurotransmitter. They are essential for the transmission of nerve impulses.

58 % (49) of the participants of my continued study reported positive changes in their mood. The exhilarating and harmonizing effect often shows already with the first dose.

- Many drugs make depressive.
- Gluttony, sweets, and lack of exercise can lead to melancholy.
- The double effect of the alga: It lifts the mood and inhibits addictive behavior.

Spirulina stops cancer growth after 3 days

In 2012, an estimated 8.2 million people died from cancer worldwide.
http://www.cancerresearchuk.org/health-professional/cancer-statistics/worldwide-cancer#heading-One

This diagnosis creates a grave crisis for those concerned. But it is no condemnation. It only wants to make us aware that we overtaxed ourselves and didn't pay enough attention to the cancer-promoting factors.

If you are diagnosed with cancer, you better increase the daily Spirulina consumption to 3 tablespoons powder and avoid all animal fats and sweets. Also, drink lots of activated water (Meyer 2015). Animal fats and sugars promote inflammation and weaken the body's defenses. Therefore, you better cut them completely out of your diet until the disappearance of any cancer cells!

We burden ourselves with radioactive rays, electromagnetic pollution, food and household chemicals. Our tap water contains heavy metals, uranium, nitrates, pesticides as well as carcinogenic and antibiotic drugs. These are not rendered harmless by the sewage plants. Using natural resources, we have the chance to cope with the morbid excrescences of civilization. In numerous studies, Spirulina proved as an excellent food remedy for cancer prevention and inhibition. Because:

The blue-green microorganism contains numerous substances with anti-cancer effect. It increases the production of tumor necrosis factor (TNF). This protein with anti-tumor effect formed by activated macrophages (large phagocytes) selectively dissolves tumor cells if not inactivated by stimulants, chemical drugs, and other toxic substances.

Even a small dose of Spirulina can have a significant healing effect as demonstrated by Babu Mathew and his team in the southernmost state of India. They gave 44 pan-tobacco chewers from Kerala who suffered from a preliminary stage of cancer of the tongue only one gram Spirulina per day. The control group of tobacco chewers received a placebo.

> In India, pan-tobacco you can get on almost every street corner. The alkaloids of this betel nut wrapped in a tobacco leaf with spicy chili sauce have a stimulating effect. During a trip to India, we tried this hot stimulant and looked like vampires. Among the Indian population, numerous jokes about the pan-tobacco chewers and their bloody cheeks are circulating.

After only one year, of the group receiving Spirulina 20 were without cancer cells. In the placebo group, only 3 had no more cancer cells! Thus it does not cost much to prevent and heal cancer!

In the early eighties was recognized that the blue protein pigment phycocyanin increases the activity of lymphocytes. These white blood cells protect against the development of tumors. In 1995, Qureshi and his team demonstrated that a water-soluble extract of Spirulina increased tumor cell killing by natural killer cells. In 2007, Roy and colleagues detected that Spirulina's phycocyanin causes the programmed cell death of liver cancer cells. The microalgae are thus suitable as a remedy for cancer in the liver. Orie Joshinari and her Japanese team from the University of Yamagata also confirmed Spirulina's liver protective effect (2013).

Because of its high beta-carotene content, researchers from Harvard University School of Dental Medicine (Dental University) in Boston tested the microorganism regarding its anti-cancer effects. In three different studies in 1986, 87 and 88 Schwartz and Shklar could prove: Spirulina reduces the number and size of tumors and slows the formation or prevents the development of cancer. The researchers concluded: An immune reaction destroyed cancerous tumors probably in the initial stage. The activated lymphocytes were T-cells (thymus-dependent lymphocytes).

Spirulina also helps with skin cancer. Since my distant relative, the music producer, writer and singer, Terry Melcher died of skin cancer, I am particularly pleased to have found this study: In May 2014, Flandiana Yogianti and her Indonesian and Japanese colleagues determined Spirulina's antitumor effect against UVB irradiation of the skin.

Recent studies have shown that Spirulina is effective against chemically induced breast cancer in rats (Ouhtit et al, 2014). And already after the third day of taking, it inhibits the dangerous pancreatic cancer (Koníčková et al. 2014; see also page 38). It would be more tolerable for humans and animals to test the side effect free microorganism especially on people without unnecessarily inflicting the animals' terrible suffering. Spirulina is approved to complement traditional drastic therapies. In this respect, it will help to protect the skin, mucous membranes, and hair. These usually suffer during chemotherapy and radiation treatment.

D. Alberts was diagnosed with lung cancer and can confirm it. His wife gave him Spirulina during his chemo and radiation therapy. Unlike other cancer patients treated with radiation Mr. A. was able to keep his weight and look better. Instead of the hard cellulose of other plants Spirulina's cell walls consist of soft, soluble mucopolysaccharides (hyaluronic acid). Therefore it is digested very fast despite the high protein content of around 60%. For the patient's inappetence, this is of advantage. Their immune system has to do enough to kill cancer cells, eliminate toxins and mobilize immune cells to fight against invading pathogens. The complex breakdown of the food into water-soluble food molecules so they can be absorbed into the watery blood plasma is another effort. We better don't require this from a sick body. By contrast, the super nutrients from the microalgae already reach the blood through the buccal mucosa, activating the healing power.

• With the diagnose cancer, deny yourself animal fats and sugars!

• Spirulina promotes the killing of tumor cells by killer cells; the blue pigment is useful as an anticancer agent in liver cancer.

• The microorganism reduces the side effects of chemos and radiation treatment. It protects the skin, mucous membranes, and hair.

• Spirulina provides the protein necessary to build muscle highly concentrated (60 %) and in an easily digestible form.

The miracle alga helps with gastritis and inflammation of the colon

Gastritis and gastric or duodenal ulcers are often caused by drugs (e. g. aspirin), alcohol or extreme stress. They manifest themselves often by nausea, vomiting and pain in the upper abdomen occurring increasingly often after eating. Treatment with proton pump inhibitors or gastric protection can lead to tiredness, dizziness, headache, insomnia, skin lesions and altered liver function tests.

https://chriskresser.com/the-dangers-of-proton-pump-inhibitors/

Mohamed M. Abdel-Daim and his Egyptian team ascertained that Spirulina is better suited for the treatment of chronic colitis than the anti-inflammatory drug sulfasalazine (Abdel-Daim et al. 2015). The anti-inflammatory alga also neutralizes acids and reduces symptoms.

The beneficial microorganism forms a protective covering in the gastrointestinal tract. Its glutamic acid ensures an acid-alkaline balance and reduces the craving for sweets and alcohol.

Both are triggers or causes of the complaints. Spirulina's high content of vitamin E reduces the stomach acid helping to relieve pain and

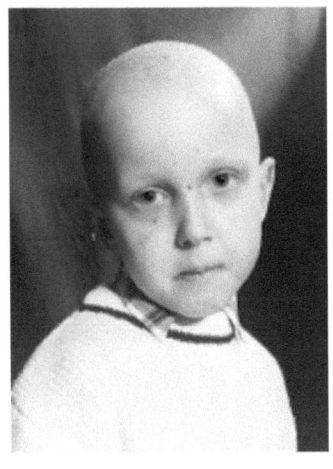 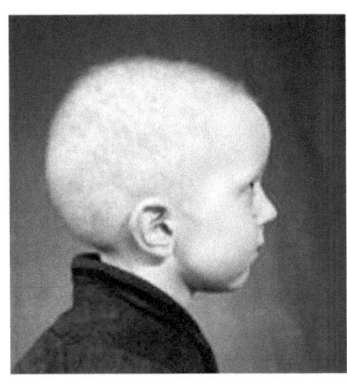 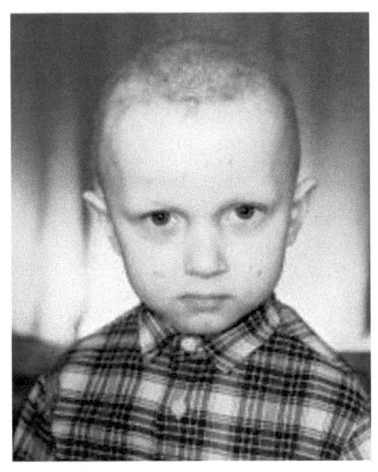

promote healing. The essential fatty acids have a beneficial effect on the healing and prevent new ulcers of the gastrointestinal tract. Spirulina's enzymes and B-complex vitamins aid digestion and reduce inflammation.

Spirulina's high iron content and vitamins B12 and folic acid cure a stomach bleeding induced by anemia.

Experience report: From 1989 to 1998, Mrs. Müller of U. suffered from stress-induced ulcers, associated with anemia. With 6 Spirulina tablets per day, she had no more complaints.

- Drugs and alcohol attack the stomach lining.
- Spirulina forms a protective lining in the gastrointestinal tract.
- The light carrier reliefs pain and inflammation.

The *Green Gold* protects the liver and kidneys

Today's diet contains too much animal protein and, therefore, harm the liver and kidneys since these organs have to process the waste products. The ammonia, formed by bacterial degradation of protein in the intestine, gets via the portal circulation to the liver. There it is degraded to urea and excreted via the kidneys. Therefore, we better avoid burdening our detoxification organs with too much animal protein. Otherwise, we could poison our gut. Acid build-up and hair loss are some of the consequences. Chemical drugs, acidifying foods and environmental toxins pollute the detoxification organs and can cause serious harm. The basic blue-green protein food buffers the excess acids in the diet and deacidifies overburdened organs. The detoxifying effect of the algae was often confirmed: 2008 by Pane and his Italian team. They tested Spirulina's absorption of cadmium and zinc and found out that the absorbency of cadmium was with 84 to 88.7% higher than that of zinc from 54.5 to 68 % essential in the diet of humans and animals. Since the algae rid the body of toxic and radioactive substances, it can prevent renal toxicity.

In 1998, Vadiraja and colleagues were able to prove that the blue pigment phycocyanin protects, among others, the liver from carbon tetrachloride. Despite Spirulina's high protein content, the uric acid increased not considerably in the blood of malnourished patients who were given 80 to 90g Spirulina per day in the Hospital Bichat in France (Santillan 1974). Also, Gitte S. Jensen and her American fellow researchers were able to demonstrate the following in a two-weeks double-blind, placebo-controlled clinical trial involving 24 people from the south of Oregon: The blue pigment phycocyanin in Spirulina improves liver function and metabolism (2016).

Zhi Huang and Zheng Winjie from China were able to show that selenium rich Spirulina is effective against liver fibrosis (2007).

In the ongoing study of currently 84 volunteers, 35 individuals improved their liver function confirming the liver regenerating and kidney detoxifying effect of the algae, though not all participants had examined their liver function. The improvement rate may be much higher.

- Large quantities of animal protein lead to acidity, hair loss and liver and kidney insufficiency.
- Spirulina buffers excess acids and protects liver and kidneys.
- The blue-green light carrier acts evidently emunctory and can thus prevent a poisoning of the excretory organs.

Spirulina protects from radiation damage

We are all surrounded by ionizing radiation without smelling or tasting it. Therefore, we better protect ourselves through the daily algae food. We prevent the accumulation of absorbed radiation energy and consequently the loss of biological function. If you take trans-continental flights, get x-rays or live near nuclear power plants you better take more Spirulina. With 10 g daily we can prevent leukemia, cataracts, heart disease, diabetes and other ailments. Countless studies with Chernobyl children confirm Spirulina's significant protective effect against gamma rays that arise in virtually all nuclear reactions. The protective effect is probably due to the stabilization of the DNA, the universal carriers of genetic information. It does not matter if we take Spirulina before or after irradiation. Fact is:

The survival food reduces the radiation dose for food contaminated with the radioactive substances cesium 137 and strontium 90.

After only a brief Spirulina consumption the urine's radioactivity decreased significantly.

In Chernobyl, Loseva and Dardynskaya administered 100 children 5 g Spirulina daily for three weeks. In this short time, the radioactivity of the urine decreased by half (1993). In Russia, Spirulina is a recognized medical food. My Bestseller *Spirulina, the Blue-Green Miracle* was also published in Russia.

Further studies can be found on my website: www.marianne-e-meyer.com

Dr. L. P. Loseva of the Scientific Research Institute of Radiation Medicine Minsk gave a 4½-year-old boy a Spirulina brand with more organically bound zinc. Since his birth, Sergei K. was suffering from food allergies. The cause was the mother's work-related lead and cadmium exposure during pregnancy. In February 1998, two months after taking Spirulina, the child's hair was sprouting for the first time in his life. Seven months later showed increased hair growth and a much-improved complexion.

- Spirulina seems to stabilizes the DNS.

- In 3 weeks, a daily dose of 5 g Spi-rulina divides the radioactivity of the urine in half.

- Before or after x-ray examinations and intercontinental flights Spirulina protects against the negative effects of harmful rays.

• With hair loss caused by cadmium and lead stress, the new hair sprouts two months after taking Spirulina.

Can Spirulina help against tinnitus?

With question mark because I also belong to the 10-15% adults who are dealing with tinnitus. The buzzing in my right ear is minor, and I prefer not to test if it will get stronger without Spirulina and the Schuessler salts 1, 3, 5, 7, 10 and 11. At the moment I try the Swedish bitters according to Maria Treben's advice: I cover the inner ear with some grease or marigold ointment (Calendula officinalis), soak two little cotton balls in Swedish bitters and stick them in the ears. Tinnitus can have many causes. It may be related to noise, stress, earwax, Candida, head or neck injuries, and ear infections. Only in a few individuals, it is a sign of a serious medical condition. We can also ease Tinnitus with reflexology. Michael Reed Gach, Ph.D. shows you some acupressure points:

http://www.acupressure.com/blog/index.php/tinnitus-ringing-ear-acupressure-points-for-the-kidneys-lower-back/

About 12 years ago, the audiologist told me, you'll just have to live with it. I recently received an email from the medical doctor in ophthalmology Dirk-Bijan Zarrinnam. He had five patients with tinnitus (acute to 2 years old). Within a few days drinking the concentrated Spirulina extract Spiruli (3 drinks per day: www.spiruli.com) they were healed. Only a patient who suffers from tinnitus for decades did not respond to Spiruli. Dr. Zarrinnam asked me for studies on this matter. I found the following online survey:

http://www.ncbi.nlm.nih.gov/pmc/articles/PMC3606192/

Juen-Haur Hwang and his Korean colleagues proved with 4 groups of 24 mice that a Spirulina water extract and its active component C-phycocyanin (C-PC) can reduce salicylate-induced tinnitus. After I had learned about this study I checked on salicylate-containing foods: Most of the vegetables, fruits, nuts, and spices I used to eat every day contain this substance, better known as aspirin! If you also want to test whether your ear noise is reduced by avoiding salicylate-containing food you can check this food list:

http://salicylatesensitivity.com/about/food-guide

Following you can order two excellent summaries on Spirulina in health management (A. Kulshreshtha et al. 2008 und M.E. Gershwin, A. Belay 2009)

www.ncbi.nlm.nih.gov/pubmed/18855693

www.researchgate.net/publication/227076610_M_E_Gershwin_A_Belay_eds_Spirulina_in_human_nutrition_and_health

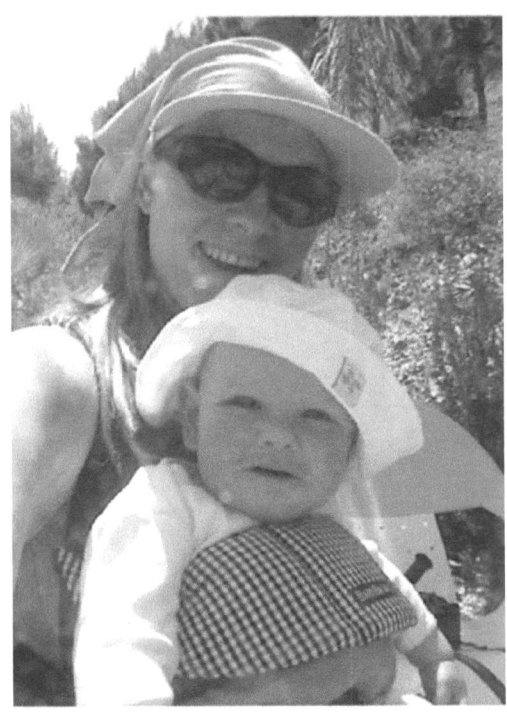

VI. WHO BENEFITS ESPECIALLY FROM SPIRULINA?

Cyanobacteria are said to have once created the oxygen atmosphere by greening the earth. Therefore we can consider them as parent substance of flora and fauna. Since all plants and animals including humans were dependent on these microorganisms, all living can benefit from Spirulina. If something is missing we, our animal friends and all plants can get it from this unique light food. Because it can store solar energy due to its blue, green and orange pigments like no other plant.

The water of Lourdes we call light water due to unusual frequencies. It contains as Spirulina the entire light spectrum of the rainbow. We depend on the sun. Therefore it is no wonder that Spirulina, the solar photons accumulator par excellence completely satisfies us, our pets and our planet.

Expectant mothers set the course for their kids' welfare

With the algae superfood, women can avoid nutrient deficiencies during pregnancy and lactation. The advantage is that Spirulina's iron, calcium, and all other nutrients are much better absorbed by the body than inorganic mineral supplements. However, because of their cleansing effect, it is better to start taking the algae half a year before pregnancy. For the detoxification process might impact the unborn child. When you desire to have children, it would be ideal if a year before the planned conception you and your partner would fill your vital fuel tank with Spirulina since it stimulates all glands. Therefore, it can stimulate the sexual glands to increase hormone secretion and improve sperm quality and quantity.

- Spirulina compensates for nutritional deficiencies during pregnancy and lactation.
- It is best for both parents to start taking Spirulina ½-1 year of procreation.

Menstruating women often suffer from iron deficiency

Women of childbearing age often suffer from iron and folic acid deficiency due to the monthly blood loss. Spirulina contains iron, folic acid and chlorophyll, vitamin B12 and other blood-forming substances. These essential elements ensure that there will be no weakness and dizziness. The regular consumption of Spirulina also eases premenstrual discomfort.

Ritalin ersatz free from side effects

Many children with ADHD have deficiencies of essential nutrients that affect the healthy development of the brain and lead to ADHD symptoms.

Struwwelpeter's hyperactivity may elicit a big grin. But if you have such a nuisance in the house, life can be hell. "The American Psychiatric Association (APA) says that 5 % of American children have ADHD. But the Centers for Disease Control and Prevention (CDC) puts the number at more than double the APA's number. The CDC says that 11 percent of American children, ages 4 to 17, have the attention disorder."

http://www.healthline.com/health/adhd/facts-statistics-infographic

I tried to find Spirulina studies on hyperactivity or ADHD. When I filled in the PubMed spacebar with "hyperactivity Spirulina" only one came up. So I assume, the compound herbal preparation (CHP) Katz et al. used at the Adaptation Clinic in Tel Hashomer, Israel, contains Spirulina. Since the alga is a proper substitute to Ritalin, Novartis may have a hand in this dispensation with the naming. The scientists conducted a randomized double-blind placebo-controlled test with 120 children newly diagnosed with ADHD or adjustment disorders. "The well-tolerated CHP demonstrated improved attention, cognition, and impulse control in the intervention group, indicating promise for ADHD treatment in children." (2010)

Countless publications on attention deficit and hyperactivity testify of the distress. 80 % of those affected are boys. They often suffer from impaired glucose tolerance and allergies. High exposure to mercury (amalgam) often acquired through breast milk or environmental toxins also burden the organism. Innumerable studies show that Spirulina reduces stress and balances mood swings and blood sugar fluctuations, promote metabolism, inhibits allergic reactions and eliminates heavy metals. The alga's essential nutrients help brain and nerve function, relaxes and provides energy and mental resilience. Therefore, Spirulina can be used as a side effect free alternative to chemical drugs such as Ritalin.

• ADHD kids are deficient in vital nutrients. Therefore the vitamin and mineral-rich algae are essential.

• Hyperactive children often suffer from poisoning and therefore respond well to the detoxifying acting, harmonizing and balancing Spirulina.

• B vitamins and alkaline minerals are calming and replace Ritalin, best used in conjunction with behavioral therapy.

Vegetarians trust Spirulina as a high-quality source of protein

The protein concentrate is particularly popular with vegans and vegetarians since it contains more than 60 % high-quality protein. Unlike protein of meat and cereal, it is promptly digested. Therefore, it does not burden the organism with the painstaking work of digestion.

Spirulina is appreciated due to a variety of nutrients and antioxidants: especially because of the vitamin B12 content. See also section "Do we need animal protein?" and "Spirulina contains active vitamin B12".

• Spirulina contains about 60 % high-quality protein and absorbable Vitamin B12.

• Spirulina's protein is easily and rapidly digested.

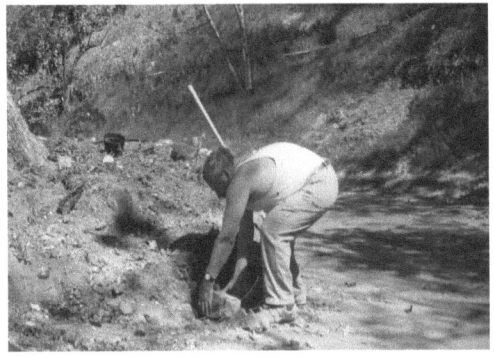

Permitted doping: power food for heavy workers and athletes

Athletes and physically hard working people need special nutrients which our usual fare today barely contains. Therefore the power food is becoming more and more popular. Athletes consume Spirulina before a sporting competition because they can count on an immediate energy boost and improved stamina. The amino acid isoleucine in Spirulina is particularly valuable: It provides energy and endurance and is involved in the repair of muscle tissue. The protein component phenylalanine helps to relieve pain and lifts the mood. Athletes especially benefit from the amino acid tryptophan: It reduces stress, balances mood swings and ensures good sleep vital before a competition. The amino acid valine is essential for athletes and heavy laborers. It provides muscle metabolism, tissue repair and maintains a nitrogen balance in the body. Spirulina's SOD and countless other enzymes as well as gamma-linolenic acid, soothe bruising and inflammation. They also prevent joint wear. In 2006, Lu and his Taiwanese team tested the effect of the algae in preventing muscle damage. 16 students took Spirulina with their normal diet for three weeks. The results on the treadmill suggest the alga prevents muscle damage and prolongs fatigue during exercise.

Athletes around the globe are already using the energizing microalgae taking 10 or more tablets ½ hour before training or competition. The Hawaiian marathoners Kawika Spaulding took 50 to 60 Spirulina tablets every day on the 3000 km route from Los Angeles to New York. Only 5 of the 14 runners arrived. During the 228 miles Hawaii marathon, the man in his mid-forties triumphed once again. Also, the storage of climber Dan Stocking from Alaska was filled with Spirulina when in 1995 he tried to conquer the highest mountain in North America, the 20,310 feet high Mt. McKinley. Spirulina contains everything the body needs for the metabolism and acts as an octane booster for the fuel in the cellular engine. Therefore, Olympians and other people dependent on performance and endurance trust the Green Gold. The South African swimmer Theo Verster achieved fantastic results with Spirulina. But initially, he took it before his meals and lost a lot of weight. After he got the advice to take Spirulina after meals he could train harder and his weight stabilized.

Several years ago, my husband and I were able to test the energy as well as stamina-giving and soreness preventing effect of Spirulina. We rolled with our rollerblades along the Zurich-Lake and burst upon 2,000 to 3,000 like-minded people who gathered for an inline-skating night. Spontaneously we decided to participate in this event.

• Spirulina is a popular concentrated power food in the athlete's scene.

• Athletes and physically hard working people use the energizing effect of Spirulina.

• The algae act like an Octane Booster for fuel in a cellular engine. Their enzymes and fatty acids lessen injuries.

• Spirulina's ideal amino acid profile soothes pains, lifts the mood, provides energy, build-up and regeneration of muscle cells and stamina.

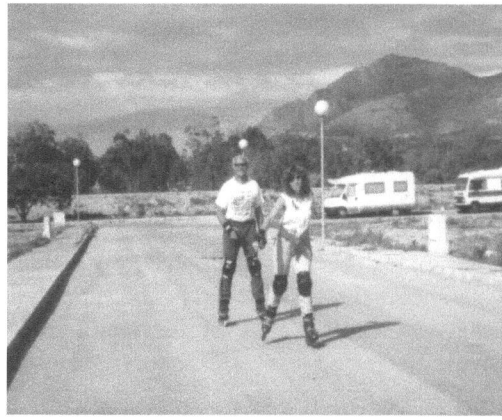

The elderly living in the fast lane again

Seniors particularly benefit from the blue-green algae, because the metabolism is slowing down with advancing age. Light foods, rich in vital substances are therefore particularly important.

In powder form, you digest Spirulina in less than an hour. Thus, the high-quality nutrients dissolve quickly in the blood and start the cell metabolism. You better don't drink soft drinks or coffee half hour before and after. The elderly who consume 5-10 g Spirulina daily, strengthen their immune system, prevent diseases, keeps the skin elastic and the hair growth and nails strong and flexible. Age spots disappear due to numerous antioxidants such as beta-carotene, vitamin E, zinc, selenium, copper, manganese, SOD, and other enzymes. With newfound energy elderly are more willing to get involved in the

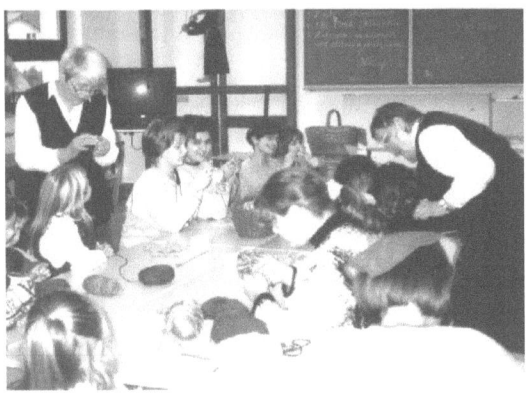

family or volunteer in the community. At age 77 my mother offered kids, as part of the AWO, a weekly needlework course and sang at age 79 publicly at the inauguration of a newly renovated temple. In her early eighties, she still participated in several dance and gymnastics groups and was on the board of the AWO. Her same-aged girlfriend (right), who often helped her with the children, learned how to use a personal computer. Occasionally she sends me an e-mail and could acquire some other interpersonal experience. She also does not want to give up her *Green Gold*. On the other hand, if we stop to get involved we risk to suffer from depression and to lead a lonely life.

Vital animals with Spirulina as a feed supplement

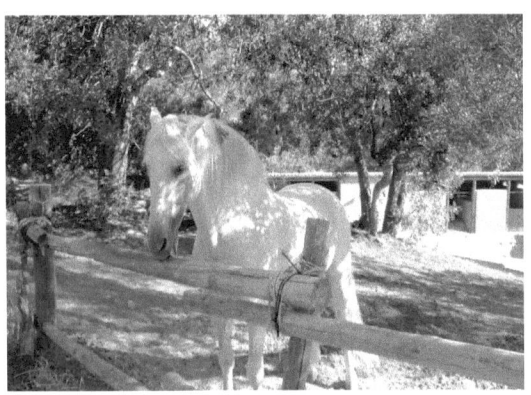

Animal breeders around the globe appreciate the microalgae as a feed additive, rich in vital substances. Because Spirulina keeps the animal's organism healthy and improves the quality of fur, skin, and feathers. It is added as a multivitamin and mineral concentrate to the fish feed and also suits as a supplemental power food for high-performance animals.

Spirulina is the insider tip for racing stable owners and horse breeders.

Our animal darlings can mostly benefit from Spirulina when arthritic afflictions occur as a result of diet sins or if the fur has lost its luster. If our pets have to travel Spirulina with all the soothing nutrients and amino acids is a suitable means to keep the excitement in borders or to help the animals to serenity.

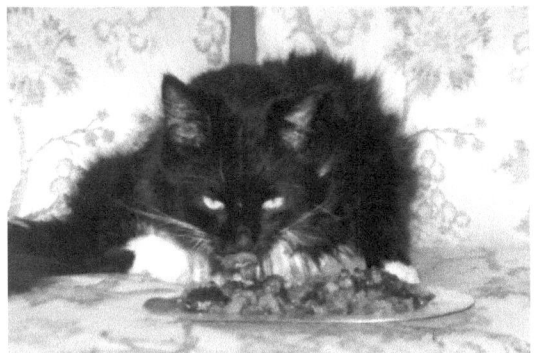

Max liked Spirulina powder scattered on wet food. He left as the 2nd oldest of our pets but the first in my arms his beautiful body.

Progress reports

In late summer 2000, the beekeeper from Östringen near Heidelberg thought to euthanize his cat because she was just lying around apathetically. Only a few months earlier, she jumped at the doorknobs and was able to move freely in the house. The apiarist heard of Spirulina from my neighbor and began to give the cat 2 x 2 Spirulina tablets daily. After only two weeks the 17-year-old velvet-pawed creature had regained its bounce and thus a bit of

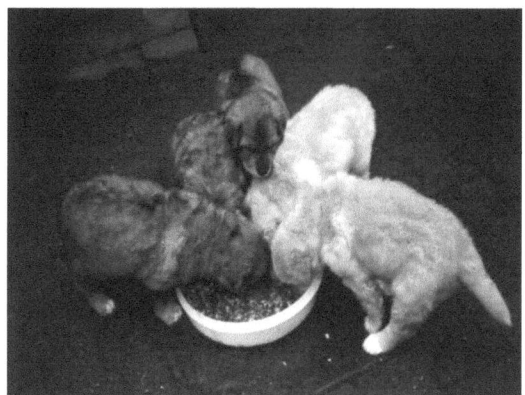

The cute Hovawart puppies pounced on their first Spirulina feed of their lives and cleaned the plate in no time

freedom, could open the doors and was the vital old cat again.

Jacky, our friend's Munsterlander suffered from severe arthritis, buckled while walking and apparently was in excruciating pain. 3 days after I had given him some Spirulina tablets several times a day he was feeling better, and his fur glistened. Two weeks later Jacky had no more symptoms, and the whole family took Spirulina from then on regularly.

Thus all living things can benefit from the microorganism as announced by the highly regarded magazine AARP with the world's largest circulation of 47 million. In its September 2005 issue, AARP described Spirulina as the most nutritious Superfood to prolong life by several years. Researchers at the Department of Rheumatology, Allergy and Clinical Immunology at the University of California at Davis determined in a 12-week study with 40 seniors that supplementing the diet with Spirulina can be a logical concept for people over 50 (or pets over 8, ed. note) who often suffer from a weak immune system or anemia (Selmi et al. 2011). See also page 56. Spirulina`s further numerous advantages, e. g., for the coronary vessels, the brain, the eyes, its anti-viral and anti-carcinogenic properties support the position of the US magazine:

Spirulina is the #1 Superfood!

VI. NATURAL BEAUTY WITH SPIRULINA

Recipes for self-made algae cosmetic

Refreshing and lifting poultice
1 teaspoon (tsp) Aloe vera gel   mix with
¼ tsp Spirulina powder

Apply to the forehead, cheeks, and neck; wash off after 10 minutes with warm water.

Anti-wrinkle plaster
1 tsp Spirulina powder   pulpify with
2 tablespoons (tbsp) olive oil

Spread on face and neck; thereover place a paper tissue and over it a damp compress towel; remove thoroughly after 20 minutes.

Skin and hair poultice
1 organic egg yolk   give dropwise
2 tbsp olive oil   to the egg
¼ tsp algae flour or   1 crushed algae tab

Work the mayonnaise in hair tips and scalp, wrap a plastic bag over it and cover with a towel. Also, apply some to the face and décolleté. After 10 minutes, remove the mask with lukewarm water. Wash the hair after 30 to 60 minutes.

A nightly 10-minute mask with ½ teaspoon Spirulina powder and subsequent coconut oil cream and some water regenerates the skin overnight.

A treat for the eyes: 2 slices of cucumber or a wet chamomile tea bags.

Tinted Moisturizer for normal skin
10 g lanolin
5g beeswax   and
3g cocoa butter   solve in a water bath; add
20 ml olive oil   and
20 Tr. Grapefruit-
seed extract   and mix; after cooling, dust
¼ tsp Spirulina powder over the cream; add
2 ml walnut shell oil   or
black tea extract (5 tsp Tea in ¼Ts boiled water) and add 3 drops perfume oil

Anti-wrinkle coconut creme
2 tbsp organic coconut oil mix with
¼ tsp Spirulina powder   and
5 drops colloidal silver   in a jar; refrigerate in summer; in other seasons, the coconut oil is solid uncooled.

Cream for a firm, full bosom
2 tbsp coconut oil   mix with
2 tbsp aloe vera gel,
1 tsp ground fennel   and
1 tsp Spirulina powder   massage a few min.

Slender and trim with the microalga

In the 1980s the Green Gold was promoted as a weight-loss wonder since Prof. E. W. Becker's study results confirmed the algae's appetite-reducing property. Nevertheless, three of my readers contacted me and claimed that taking Spirulina would trigger cravings. Reasons could be the lack of nutrients by an unbalanced diet or drugs, sugar, cigarette or alcohol consumption. In such cases, a radical cleansing of the colon is recommended (see page 27). Because with slagged intestinal walls the valuable substances of the algae can not be absorbed and supplied to the blood. Only when the crusty deposits are dissolved and eliminated, we can start the reducing diet. Otherwise, we only produce expensive urine and feces!

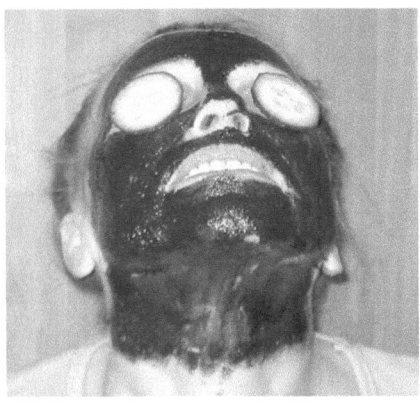

Spirulina helps with cellulite

The orange peel skin is a common problem usually in girls and women. We eat more and more fats and sweets but instead of compensating with physical exertion many females turn into couch potatoes, often resulting in lymphatic congestion and mild edema. How can you get rid of already existing bumps and prevent new ones? You could stir 1 tablespoon of psyllium husk powder in ½ l cranberry juice and drink it twice a day or eat it as pudding. Also:

A low-fat diet that includes plenty of niacin and a combination of massage with firming gel, bike riding, jogging, trampoline jumping and stretching exercises help to smooth the skin.

You can also test the following anti-cellulite workout:

https://www.youtube.com/watch?v=2Hp-B2UhG4rM

Niacin (Vitamin B3) accelerates fat burning. Yeast, brown, red, and green algae, pollen, grass juice, rice hulls, mushrooms, fish, poultry, and meat contain this vitamin. 10-15 g Spirulina already covers the entire daily requirement. Niacin ensures good blood circulation and healthy skin explaining why vegetarians have sometimes no rosy skin and look unhealthy. However, the exterior is deceiving.

Firming gel: Mix ½ tsp Spirulina powder with 1 tsp aloe vera gel and 1 tbsp soy oil. Spread evenly on both hands and apply to the affected areas on the inner rear thigh. Streak upward with bent knees and hands behind the knees. Again squat and repeat smoothing out 15 to 20 times. After ten minutes wash off the dried thigh mask with warm water and finish with cold showers.

VII. SPIRULINA EXPERIENCES AROUND THE WORLD

In more than forty countries Spirulina is offered in the form of tablets, capsules or powder, or added to foods, beverages, and cosmetics. In the late 70s began in Japan the sale of blue-green algae. In 1979, the company Earthrise Farms introduced the algae in health food stores in the US and distributed them equally on multidimensional sales level by the company Light Force (Henrikson 1997). In 1981, the heading of the tabloid National Enquirer from June 1 on this medically recommended anorectic, initiated a real sell-off in the US which also spilled across the pond to Europe. But since few Spirulina farms were productive at that time, the dealers could not get the algae delivered in the desired quantities. They mixed in large amounts of cheap green fillers, such as alfalfa grass. Of course, the people felt cheated; mainly because they took Spirulina for a magic pill for losing weight and expected a quick success.

Since 1987, the algae again experiences a comeback with a rising trend since 1991, at around 30 to 40 percent.

Result reports from Germany

The Hippocratic Oath which requires medics never to harm the patients is still taken very seriously by some doctors, I was told by a Berliner living in Battenberg. She had no **hair due to chemotherapy**. I advised her Spirulina and later learned that her hair immediately began to sprout fully after taking the algae. She showed her doctor my book. He was very excited and recommends Spirulina ever since! Fortunately, there are still those doctors. But many give Spirulina to their family members but prescribe their patients chemical drugs.

Mrs. C. of I. suffered from intestinal problems due to a **yeast infection**. Her alternative practitioner advised her to take Spirulina. After a few days, Mrs. C. was well, and the fungal infection was no longer an issue.

After 5 months of taking Spirulina, Mr. S. from N. had **no more use for glasses**. He had no more colds and his energy increased.

Mrs. I. from N. was suffering from an **autoimmune disease**. She could hardly eat anything. Taking daily 3 x 1 teaspoon Spirulina powder in apple or pineapple juice, the body got the required protein and all the minerals and vitamins. Mrs. I. thinks she would not be alive anymore without Spirulina.

Mrs. K. from E. often suffers from **nasal congestion**. Whenever she swallows 3 or 4 Spirulina tabs she feels better within minutes.

Mr. W. from Sch. suffered from **hay fever** every year. Since he takes Spirulina as a food supplement, he is free of symptoms.

Mrs. B. from W. had after showering a generalized **itching**. She tried various soaps, shower gels and various mild and pH-neutral washing lotions. But the itching always remained the same. After taking Spirulina, Mrs. B. had no more skin problems after showering or bathing.

Mrs. P. from W. has suffered no **cold sore** since the regular use of the cyanobacteria.

Mrs. R. from E. had for years a **goiter**. With Spirulina she now has no more problems with the thyroid. Her cat is crazy about the algae tabs.

Mrs. M. from U. suffered from **anemia**, caused by stomach ulcers. Between 1989 and 1998, she came down with it twice a year. She took 6 Spirulina tablets daily. Shortly after her blood values were excellent and she was free of stomach discomfort. As a side-effect, she has flexible, beautiful fingernails and shiny, soft hair.

I advised Mrs. S. from M. to regularly take Spirulina. A few weeks later, she told me she could **sleep** soundly and had no more problems turning over in her mind during sleepless phases. Also, the **concerns** during the day did no longer depress her. Her dry skin and the calluses on the feet were gone. The desire for meat and alcohol beverages had subsided, and the **craving** for fruits, greens, and raw vegetables increased. Mr. S. was finally able to **sleep** once again after a long time. His already changed **age spots** faded and got smaller, some completely disappeared.

The competent beekeeper who offers every Saturday his bee products on the market in Heidelberg is excited by the light food. On his 17-year-old cat, he learned about Spirulina's effect. With young children, animals, and plants the healing effects can be well tested since they can not imagine improvements. See page 68, chapter *Vital animals with Spirulina as a feed supplement*. The woman of the beekeeper had a **hip replacement** surgery coming up. She could hardly sleep at night with groaning and got up only at noon. When she began to take Spirulina, the pain eased. Mrs. B. was able to sleep again at night and could meet her domestic duties in the morning. The family atmosphere relaxed because the husband was not kept awake by the groans of his wife and had no more to suffer from lack of care.

Mrs. W. from E. suffered for a long time from **neurodermatitis** relapses that occurred every 3 to 4 weeks. In a health food store, she got Spirulina recommended in increasing doses. Mrs. W. took 2-4 Spirulina tablets daily. When she came into the store three days later, the reddish scaly rash on the face was barely visible.

Mrs. K. from M. reported that Spirulina brought her **hot flashes** during menopause to disappear. Mr. K. had several surgeries on his spine. The former truck driver took 3 x 1 Tramal Long 100, 3 x 40 drops Valoron® and 3 x 25 drops Novalgin for his **backache**. On his birthday I gave him a big glass of Spirulina tablets. He sorted them into his pillbox and took daily 3 x 2. A few weeks later I called him. We talked about my book on water. I said, our drinking water contains traces of drugs that are excreted in the urine and not eliminated from the treatment plants. But not from me, he said. Since I take Spirulina, I no longer need medication. If you consider that Tramal is quite a gun, I would call that a miracle. Imagine how pure our drinking water could be if all people would take Spirulina against health problems!

Do you, my dear readers, still believe in coincidences? On 18.7.16, I looked in vain for my file letters from readers and checked my e-mails for the success stories of my readers. Lo and behold, a new e-mail with more experience reports: Mrs. S. from K. could stop with Spirulina her incipient **hip and knee problems**. Her father had a **Guillain-Barre syndrome** at age 85. She nursed him 1½ years. Mrs. S. administered her father Spirulina and OPC. After 6 months he returned slowly to his feet though the doctors gave him no hope that he would ever be mobile again. He reached an age of nearly 94 years. Mrs. S. recommended a fellow patient Spirulina who then got rid of her yearlong **irritable bowel syndrome**. Her brother (my own is, unfortunately, resistant to advice) could hardly eat anything after taking **chemo** tablets. He had lost 7 kg. After a few weeks of taking Spirulina he had his appetite back and tolerated the chemotherapy tablets.

This reminds me painfully of my girlfriend Gertrude who after chemo for stomach cancer left her emaciated, tormented body in June 1994. Unfortunately only a few months later I learned about the value of Spirulina. Perhaps Gertrude would be still alive today. In my autobiographical novel *Doris Day and my Search for Relatives* I memorialized Gertrude, and I hope that many readers can learn from what she had left us.

Success stories from other countries

Many doctors and pharmacists in South Africa recommend Spirulina against infections and weak resistance. Perhaps this is the reason why the pharmaceutical industry reduces prices of their AIDS drugs there. The much cheaper algae could outdo them otherwise. In South Africa Spirulina's popularity is caused by the Talk programs of East Coast Radio. The station conducts regular interviews about health products. As manager of a wholesale with such products, Estie Schreiber got active replies of her conversation about Spirulina. Thanks to Marcus Rohrer I was able to read dozens of these letters. From these experiences of users, we can draw conclusions. Estie was also not immune to the cruel excesses of civilization. Her perfectionism left her with all the tasks as a mother of two small children and the frantic work in the company no time for herself. I was a perfectionist, black, and white, right and wrong ... somehow I was a machine eating health-food. She became aware of this after having been **overthrown in the depths of despair by the diagnosis of cancer.** The nagging questions came and then suddenly, like a single bright ray of sunshine through the dark overcast sky, she realized: The microalgae in her product range combines all the colors of the spectrum in itself and will be right for her since many researchers proved their ability to promote well-being. Mrs. Schreiber transferred this philosophy to her live and could now after two years lived to the fullest assess: I have a rainbow in my life, I'm so happy and satisfied. Also, a young woman from Wartburg who was stressed by family and career and went to night school 6 days a week wrote: One month ago I discovered Spirulina, and now I can take on the world. **No more yawning at work, no more screaming with the family** when I come home. My job is less stressful. Now, on Saturday mornings I am awake at my lectures and have much **more energy**.

Mrs. S. P. from Durban also felt so **energized** after three months of taking Spirulina that my husband can not rival with me if you know what I mean. One thing was unclear to her: Why can not the insurance company pay for such a good product? If more people would take Spirulina, they'd have less often sought medical attention. Healthier members mean fewer demands on medical services. Yes, it would be nice if conflicts of interest would not be standing the way of the change from the disease business to the health care business. But the people earning from diseases would rather ban Spirulina and other natural remedies.

The daughter of Mrs. P. was on her wedding day crying, nervous and full of anxiety. The hairdresser and the makeup woman waited. Eventually, Spirulina came into Mrs. P.'s mind. She gave her daughter two tablets. Ten minutes later she was a different person. She was calm and composed. Her tension and nervousness were gone. All wedding guests said they had never seen such a radiant bride.

Mrs. M. U. of Wolmaransstad needed anti-inflammatory pills against rheumatic pains. The women in the pharmacy recommended Spirulina. Since then the 55-year-old woman had no more pain.

The 66-year-old Mrs. V. R. from Bloemfontein suffered from cancer and severe pain. 2½ years ago her uterus was removed. In November 1999 were still cancer cells found in her body. I was devastated, this horrific death sentence that is admeasured to you so mercilessly. On the radio, she heard of Spirulina and bought a bottle. Now I have a new strength. I no longer suffer from pain and therefore do not need painkillers. I am a new person! And I even lost weight!

A 67-year-old man from Pretoria writes: Since 5 years, I am divorced due to **impotence** and have spent thousands of rands to be all right but to no avail. I heard of Spirulina and bought a bottle. In the first 2 days, I took 1 tablet daily. In the next 2 days, I took 2 and then 3 tablets. That was on January 13, 2000. In the night of January 18, I woke up with such a shock about my erect penis that I was so overjoyed and kissed the Spirulina bottle.

Shortly after surgery, Mrs. D. from Despatch had only weak defenses and picked up an **infection** under the fingernails. Half a year after she tried Spirulina she was a member of a hiking club. She could sleep better than ever. Her hair, nails, and skin improved noticeably: Everyone has noticed that I look better and feel better. Nobody believes me that I am 63 years old.

Mrs. S. D. T. suffered from a degenerative disease. She could not get up in the morning. Hugely embarrassing was her **forgetfulness**. After two years of taking Spirulina, she was fit again with her memory working great. She thinks she is the living proof of the effect of the algae because *my doctor had told my husband that I would never be able to live a normal life. I not only lead a normal life but a better quality life than ever before.*

For 15 years, Mrs. M. S. from Witbank suffered under extremely **intense itching** on the feet. No drug and no doctor were able to help. When she heard of Spirulina, she had just once again suffered an associated inflammation of the sinuses and tried it. Within three months her immune system strengthened and her feet completely healed.

L. S. writes: Only if you stop taking Spirulina you recognize the benefits.

The life of the student K. R. had changed completely after taking Spirulina. For the first time, he slept the night before an examination. He had more energy than ever, a better concentration and he was **no longer anxious.**

Mrs. E. W. from Durban calls Spirulina the miracle supplement of the millennium since it prevents cancer, checks weight, regulates digestion and gives the body the chance to preserve its youthfulness and vitality.

Mrs. K. B., a 37-year-old Swiss native was a diabetic all her life. In 1995 she suffered from **kidney failure** noticeable by fluid retention and related weight gain. Her blood pressure was too high and renal function only at 25 %. At the end of 1999, two physicians suggested a kidney transplant. In early 1999, she tried Spirulina. Only 2 tabs per day increased her kidney function while the blood sugar level dropped. A kidney transplant was no longer a consideration.

Mr. L. of Link Hills suffered from **hypertension** since his youth. In January 1999, he began to take Spirulina. In spring his blood pressure was with 129/76 in the normal range. His chronic insomnia had an end, also taking sleeping pills and antidepressants.

Mrs. J. J. from Durban had heard that Spirulina heals internally, fights infections and strengthens the defenses. Since she intended breast surgery, she took 6 Spirulina tabs daily to build her resistance. A week after surgery, her plastic surgeon said in all the years of his practice he had never seen someone whose scars had healed so quickly.

Mrs. H. N. of Helen, Georgia overcame her chronic **fatigue** syndrome thanks to Spirulina.

Mrs. M.S. from Fullerton in California suffered from Reiter's disease, a painful form of **arthritis**. Since many analgesics cause an upset stomach, a girlfriend gave her Spirulina. After a few days, something wonderful happened: I realized I had no pain. She didn't trace it back to Spirulina but to a natural cause. A few weeks after her stock of the algae tablets was running out, the excruciating pain returned. After a few painful days, she remembered it must have been the Spirulina after all and got herself another glass. Shortly after re-taking arthritis ceased and Mrs. S.'s other mental and physical condition had improved.

The 63-year-old Mrs. A. W. of Melbourne in Florida had severe pain in her fingers and ankles. Three weeks after taking Spirulina, the **soreness and pain** vanished. After the second bottle, Mrs. W. could work eight or more hours at a time (cleaning) without having pain. Two weeks after she had discontinued taking Spirulina the pain returned. Taking Spirulina again, the swelling and pain disappeared. Some of my study participants had the same experience. It usually takes 1 to 3 weeks until the pain ends. After withdrawing it comes back after 2 to 3 weeks. But in re-taking, it ceases after 3 to 5 days.

Since Mrs. C.B.L. from Indialantic, Florida, takes Spirulina she has a lot more energy, is not **hungry between meals** and has no more colds and flues.

Mrs. R. from L.A. had a **goiter**. Since the regular algae diet her thyroid functions normally and the goiter is gone. Like experiences had my mother's niece, Karin Riesinger and my mother's sister, Anneliese Umbreit.

By the way, if you are a fan you can read more about my famous relative, Doris Day than you find in tabloids. This book (the new edition's title will be *Family Code*) I gave her for her 90th birthday:

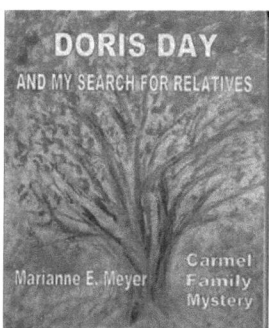

VIII. RESULTS OF THE ONGOING SPIRULINA STUDY

The 84 participants who have to date filled out the questionnaire suffer from various immunodeficiency diseases such as AIDS, acne, allergy, anemia, arthritis, candida, chronic bronchitis, other inflammatory conditions, depression, diabetes, herpes, heart problems, cancer, circulatory problems, hepatobiliary disorders, stomach and intestinal ulcers, eczema, osteoporosis, rheumatism, sarcoidosis, thyroid problems and psoriasis. Their suffering was mainly caused by the acidity of their humor. The study aims to assess Spirulina's impact on making destructive chemicals, scalpels and harmful rays redundant.

> *Working hypothesis: Malaise develops due to unnatural lifestyle, diet, and environmental factors gradually into the disease. The immune potentiating blue-green microalgae Spirulina regenerate the organism within 4 to 6 months.*
>
> *Health disorders indicate poisoning of the body and the effort to get rid of anything unusual. The only meaningful therapy is, therefore, to help the overburdened organism with the excretion of acids. To eliminate the acid crystals, do a one-week fasting with activated water and, if desired, with the juice of fresh lemons and ½ teaspoon of honey. Fresh vegetable and fruit juices or water-containing fruits and veggies also help to detoxify. Fruits contain living, structured water with the power to dissolve and flush contaminants. Only when water forms crystals, so-called clusters, it can fulfill its role as a solvent and purify the body. Our tap water is treated to death and only able to revive if we use a water activator (Meyer 2015 or DrMarianneEMeyer @ gmail.com for a PDF file).*

The Participants in the study were asked to consume at least 10 g Spirulina (one tablespoon algae powder or 20 to 25 tablets) 4 to 6 weeks daily. After this time, they could the rich in vital substances helical pipsqueak certify different positive effects on their health. Following the improvements of body functions, symptoms or laboratory values in percentages recorded by the subjects. The multiple answers of the 84 persons indicate a harmonizing and balancing effect of microalgae on the organism.

Improvements by taking Spirulina

Immune function •	63% (53 persons)
Excretion	60.7% (51 persons)
Mood	58% (49 persons)
Relaxation / Sleep	52.4% (44 persons)
Digestive	52.4% (44 persons)
Skin	51% (43 persons)
Energy and endurance	51% (43 persons)
Altered diet	45% (38 persons)
Pain	41.7% (35 persons)
Liver function reading	41.5% (35 persons)
Memory performance	40.5% (34 persons)
Circulation	35% (29 persons)
Allergic reactions	35% (29 persons)
Blood value, anemia	31% (26 persons)
Inflammation	27% (23 persons)
Blood sugar	22,5% (19 persons)
Blood Pressure	22.5% (19 persons)
Eyes	22.5% (19 persons)
Cholesterol	21.4% (18 persons)
Hair	18% (15 persons)

(• fewer infections, mouth ulcers, warts, fungus, herpes and other signs of immunodeficiency)

The investigation showed: The subjects were able to achieve improvements in their health status with the blue-green microalgae, regardless of their diet and lifestyle.

The indirect questioning by individually completed questionnaires may have only a tendentious significance. For example, only those people could make a statement about their liver values or general blood counts who had performed laboratory tests. It would be interesting to have status reports conducted for all participants before and after taking Spirulina. Several volunteers answered only some of the questions.

A more detailed review I had hoped to get after a charity biking tour which is performed in Germany every year for kids with cancer. On August 17, 2001, I joined the celeb bikers for about 20 kilometers and donated 10 large glasses of Spirulina for the partaking oncologists. When I ordered the 10 glasses, the supplier was fond of the idea, wanting to supply us with any required amount of algae tablets for free. Other vendors are also convinced of their products and are donating them for study purposes. In Russia, India, Africa and other countries, the tests are carried out on children. But my study efforts fell by the wayside. One of the professors was never reachable. Another took around 40 minutes to steal my time making fun of my idealism and shocking me by saying: I do not believe in preventive medicine, we need cancer because of overpopulation! He also denied me to send the algae food to the parents, so I gave up. He said you first should prove whether this miracle food works. Why, are the countless international studies not satisfying as evidence?

The cancer specialist had neither read my book nor the seven pages of references I had sent him before. These independent studies from around the world document Spirulina's effect against cancer. Hopefully, in the future, many more clinical trials are carried out because every year hundreds of thousands of people are given up by doctors when they are at their wits' end. It would be a blessing for mankind and in the spirit of Hippocrates when the proven immune-boosting microalgae are given to the patients with so-called hopeless cases of cancer.

Likewise, it would avoid bad karma if scientists try Spirulina's anti-cancer effects more often in clinical human studies instead of mistreating mice and hamsters with poison. Of course, the disease industry only benefits from man-made drugs and are not amused about Spirulina as a research object. And members of the caste of the politicians who are on the industry's drip-feed couldn't care less either.

So it is up to us to carry out these investigations. How? Very easily:

Go to the doctor, get your blood values and a copy of the results. A year after taking Spirulina check your blood again, compare both and draw conclusions.

As in chapter *What reactions may occur?* mentioned due to the strong cleansing effect of the algae, you may have more or less severe reactions. Some participants had long forgotten complaints on short notice. These were mainly pain in the joints and blemishes such as pimples and blackheads. Other effects of the cleansing process are sweating, diarrhea and increased amounts of urine.

Many of the 84 subjects who made the following observations while taking Spirulina had two or more symptoms of elimination:

Sweats 17
Diarrhea 15
Nausea 12
Bloating 10
Constipation 11
Alternating diarrhea & constipation 10
Circulation problems / vertigo 7
Increased appetite 7
Appetite decrease 9
Lesions 9
Increasing volume of urine 6
Joint pain 6
Herpes simplex infection (cold sores) 5

Spirulina in combination with drugs

According to the data, participants frequently treated with penicillin, sulfonamide and corticosteroids have significant immune deficiencies.

In 12 of the 14 anemic participants who regularly take anti-inflammatory drugs, after four to six weeks of consuming Spirulina, the blood values improved so much that the hemoglobin level was in the normal range. In 35 subjects the liver function reading was tested; all showed improvements. Thus, the alga's detoxifying and regenerating effect can be certified. Therefore it can be used in combination with chemotherapy and radiation treatment.

8 of 17 subjects suffering from cancer consumed the microalgae during chemotherapy and could confirm that it protects skin, mucous membranes, and hair. Thus, Spirulina ensures that the side effects of traditional therapeutic measures are within tolerable limits.

Spirulina related to nutrition and lifestyle

Almost half of participants (49%) mostly live off cereals, bread, potatoes, vegetables, salad, fish, and poultry. Frequently consumed snacks are fruit, yogurt, cake, and energy bars. 23 subjects eat up to four times a week fast foods such as hamburger, pizza, sausages and roast chicken. They regularly enjoy ice cream or coffee cakes. In this group, fewer fruits, salads, and vegetables were eaten as the nutrition societies recommend, but lots of bread with sausage or cheese and dairy products. They consumed too many fats, sweets, and salts.

14 subjects consumed vegetarian wholefoods such as cereal mush (primarily millet, buckwheat, and spelt), vegetables, salad, and fruit. 7 participants ate additional natural yogurt, cheese, and free-range eggs.

Only 18 people exercise daily a half to one hour (jogging, walking, aerobics, cycling). 16 move three times weekly, 16 twice and 25 once per week. 11 did not specify.

Astonishing result: All subjects achieved positive effects with Spirulina, regardless of their lifestyle and nutrition. However, whether this means you need not change your lifestyle and eating habits, you will better find out for yourself. In any case, I wish you on your way into the light all the best! I would be happy if I did succeed in inspiring you to lead a happy and healthy life. If you have more faith in the self-healing powers of your body, you need not fear any epidemics.

With any health problem, just thank for the perfect body, with which the creation has equipped you and ask what your body needs to function optimally. Have I enough fresh air, the sun, pure water and exercise granted to allow the juices to flow? Did I rest, leisure and sleep to provide for regeneration?

When you fill out the following questionnaire and send it, preferably by e-mail, I'll send you one of my books with a personal dedication. You can find them on my website:

www.marianne-e-meyer.com

Particularly noteworthy are the Spirulina experiences of health expert Halima Neumann who in the mid-1990s introduced me to the beneficial microalgae. A considerable part of the questionnaires for my ongoing Spirulina study she kindly let her seminar participants fill out. During Halima's more than twenty years of seminar work with cancer patients she found out:

The effectiveness of all natural substances including blue-green algae achieved a particularly rapid and sustained healing success of my participants when they at the same time changed their diet in terms of detoxification and deacidification.

In the new edition of her book *"Stopp Krebs"* Halima Neumann writes:

More than 30 years ago I conducted an anticancer part fasting, in Hawaii building up my exhausted body with daily 30 g Spirulina powder. I distributed the amount over two meals with the addition of coconut water. The treatment consisted mainly of the juice of green papaya, fresh coconut water, noni fruits and of chewing barley grass. With fatigue and nocturnal food cravings, a 3rd Spirulina portion was always an immediate remedy and provided a pleasant, all around good feeling.

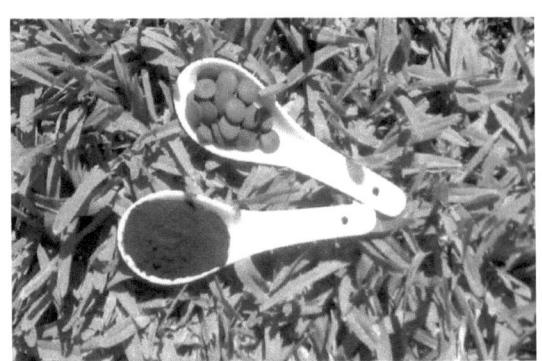

IV. HOW TO USE SPIRULINA IN THE KITCHEN

To slowly get used to the seaweed flavor we initially better use Spirulina with foods and spices covering it such as apples, bananas, plums, pineapple, ginger, cucumbers, onions, horseradish, and celery.

In the mid-1990's Halima Neumann had visited me in L. A. She introduced me to a wellness drink with 1 large banana, 1 apple, 5 to 6 dates, 1 tablespoon of Spirulina and a cup of water liquefied in a blender. It tasted so good that for long I used this as a breakfast substitute. After that, I could suck the Spirulina tablets like candy.

Powdered Spirulina you better stir with just a little water as you make a sauce with flour, otherwise, it forms clumps. Sprinkling the algae flour on purees, soups or vegetable dishes it binds well and does not thread like other algae. Here is a trick on how we can easily stir Spirulina powder into liquids: Mix it with whey, millet, almond powder or coconut flakes. The easiest Spirulina dish is a finished apple puree, in which we stir 1 to 2 tsp algae powder with a fork.

My current favorite and very quick dish with Spirulina is this:

I wash 1 fresh fig, break it up, dent it and insert ½ tsp Spirulina powder. Kneading the outside helps to mix the green flour with the flesh of the fig.

Almost as fast you can press the powder with a fork into a banana.

Recipes

Flavorful meals

Teaspoon	tsp
Tablespoon	tbsp
Drop	dr
Ground	gr
Small	sm
Large	lg
Handful	hf
Pinch	pi

Bean burger

Brown 1 onion in a pan; add 2 cloves of garlic &	
½ tsp salt	add
1 cup of beans	cooked or canned, drain, thicken with
1 tsp psyllium powder	or 2-3 tbsp oatmeal, flavor with
herbal spices & pepper;	form a patty; fry it, cut
1 wholewheat roll	in half; spread it with a
½ tsp Spirulina flour	mixed with
½ tsp mustard	and
1 tsp organic ketchup	top the roll with the burger and the onions, add
tomato & cucumber	slices and a lettuce leaf

Chicory salad

2 chicory plants	clean & cut in broad stripes
1 slice pineapple	peel, dice, add to chicory
½ avocado	mash with a fork, add
1 tsp Spirulina flour	
½ tsp salt, herbs	and
1 pi cayenne powder	and spread over the chicory

If you do not like avocados, you can use walnut or almond butter or sesame or walnut oil.

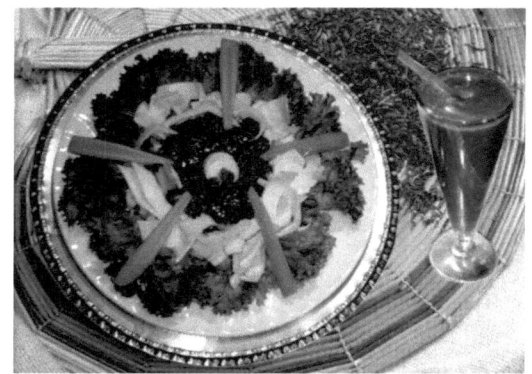

Pea puree

250 g young peas	from the shell, or
1 sm can *extra fine*	mix with the flesh of
8 olives	or 1 avocado
1 tsp Spirulina flour	
1 clove garlic	
1 sm jalapeno pepper	and
½ tsp sea or rock salt	in a blender

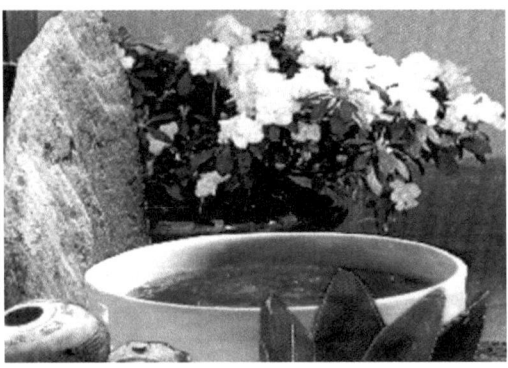

Use the puree as spread or dip garnished with raw vegetable strips on any buffet. Or serve as an accompaniment to vegetable dishes.

Green onion salad

2-3 green onions	clean; cut cross 2-3 times then in longitudinal stripes
1 zucchini	cut in 3 parts and lengthwise in stripes; braise lightly 5 minutes in butter, allow cooling; stir
2 tbsp Olivenöl	with
1 tsp Spirulina fl.	and
a little Wasser	until smooth; mash
1 glove of garlic	with finely chopped basil and thyme
½ tsp sea salt licorice powder	in salad dressing and 1 pi or stevia if you like it sweet; spread the sauce over the vegetables; cut
½ red jalapeno	in tiny pieces and sprinkle over the salad

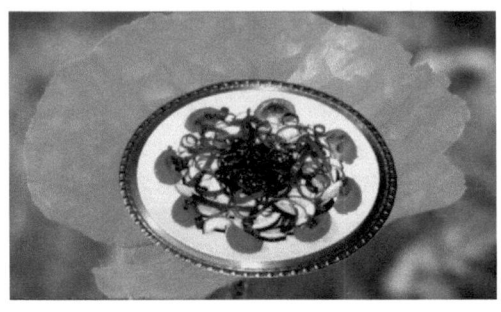

Stewed vegetables with rice

1 cup of brown rice	or parboiled, bring with
2 cups of water	to a boil and simmer gently; steam chopped
1 lg onion,	
1 red bell pepper,	
1 eggplant	in little water; spice with
sea salt & cayenne	add
4 tsp olive oil	(cold-pressed); allow to cool a little; sprinkle
1 tsp Spirulina flour	over each plate

Ginger sesame spread

1 tbsp Spirulina flour	mix with
4 tbsp applesauce	and a little water
½ tbsp ginger powder	or rasp a thumb-sized piece of ginger
40 g ground sesame	and
3 tbsp sweet whey powder; season with salt & lemon	

You can use this delicious paste, like any other spreads listed, as a dip or base for salad dressings, sauces, soups, and stews.

Chickpeas with "peanut" dressing

1 cup chickpeas	soak overnight and cook gently for 30 minutes; stir
3 tbsp soy flour	with
5 tbsp sesame oil	until smooth; add
1 tsp Spirulina	squeeze
1 clove of garlic	through a garlic press
1 sm onion	chop finely; add

½ tsp herbal salt
½ tsp ginger   or fennel powder and spread the dressing over the peas. Best side dishes: quinoa, rice, and polenta

Chickpea pie with avocado sauce

2 cups pea flour   mix with
6 tbsp coconut oil   (possibly flavor neutral*)
100 g goat's cheese   (or Parmesan), crumble,
1 egg   and
½ tsp salt   in a bowl, work into a smooth dough; place in the refrigerator for half an hour; meanwhile wash
1 red pepper
1 eggplant   and
1 zucchini   and dice roughly
2 onions   peel, divide into eighth and mix with
3 eggs
1 cup of cream
2 tsp oregano
1 tsp vegetable broth powder and
½ tsp of pepper   in a blender

fill 2/3 of the dough into a greased springform or casserole, roll out the rest and cut into ½ inch wide strips; add the vegetables and cover with the strips; bake in oven at 90°C 1½ hours (or 20 min. at 175 °C).

For the sauce mash the meat of

1 avocado   with
5 tbsp coconut oil   (flavor neutral)
1 tsp Spirulina flour
salt and pepper   with a fork

*) www.foodrenegade.com/how-to-choose-a-good-coconut-oil

Coriander ground patties (vegan)

2 tbsp chia seeds   soak in 6 tbsp water
400 g chickpeas   fresh cooked or canned drain in a sieve
1 large onion   finely dice
1 garlic clove   chop finely
1 bunch coriander   mince finely; leave 2 stalks; season the chickpeas with cumin, salt & pepper   and puree finely; knead in the onion-garlic mixture, chia seeds & coriander. Season to taste. With moistened hands form 5-6 patties and bake with 4 tbsp coconut oil 2 minutes per side.

Lentil noodles with mushroom paste

100 g fresh or 10 g dried mushrooms; cook in
½ l water   for 7 minutes
5 tbsp red lentils   mill in coffee grinder, add and simmer for 4 minutes
1-2 onions   finely dice; steam in
1 tbsp coconut oil   until golden; put the pasta water   on the stove; cook
90 g lentil noodles   or garbanzo noodles as directed; alternatively you can make the lentil noodles yourself:
2 tbsp chia seeds   soak ½ hour in 8 tbsp water or use 1-2 eggs; grind
200 g lentils   add
2 tbsp water   with the chia mash work until you get a crumbly dough.

It is best to use the noodles with a pasta machine. But you can also roll them out and cut them yourself, or create a crumble soup from the whole.

Spicy Porridge

1 l water, broth or   oatmeal milk bring to a boil; stir in
8 tbsp of oatmeal   or spelt flakes; let simmer for 5-7 minutes; add
1 cup green veggies   (peas, leeks, zucchini) and
1 cup of yellow "   (carrots, pumpkin, corn) simmer for further 7-9 minutes and let cool a little; season with salt & cayenne pepper stir in
1 tbsp Spirulina flour and upgrade with
1 tbsp seeds   (sunflower, pumpkin)

Red lentil spread

½ l veggie broth	bring to a boil; finely chop
1-2 onions	and steam until golden in
1 tbsp coconut oil	mill
5 tbsp of lentils	in a coffee grinder and stir in the vegetable broth; simmer for 5 min., then add
1 tbsp sea salt	or vegetable broth powder and add the onions; you can thicken it with
1-2 tsp psyllium husk powder; season with salt & pepper	and
1 tbsp	lemon juice; let cool a little and stir in

1 tbsp Spirulina flour and store in a jar in the refrigerator; you can upgrade with 2 tsp of germinated sunflower seeds

Pesto for the respiratory system

1 bunch plantain	gather on the meadow, mix with
½ cup camelina	or hemp oil,
1 tsp ginger,	fennel or anise and
½ tsp sea salt	liquefy in blender; fill in a screw top jar; thicken with

1 tbsp Spirulina fl. refine with organic lemon juice

Leftover pancakes (gluten free)

3 tbsp chia seeds	soak ½ hour in
½ cup of water	(or 3 eggs) mix with
rice or potato puree	leftover and
rice or millet flour	depending on the amount of the rice or puree; add
½-1 tsp sea salt	
½ tsp bicarb	and
2 cups of rice milk	if necessary more or less stir out all ingredients and

bake them from both sides in a pan with some coconut oil.

1 lg onion	mince and steam golden in
1 tbsp coconut oil	
1 clove of garlic	mince and cook with
100 g mushrooms	e. g., shiitake, champignon; fry until the liquid is evaporated; add
1 tsp tomato paste	and
3-4 tbsp	coconut cream; season with
sea salt & pepper	mix and add
1 tsp Spirulina fl.	with

1 tsp veggie broth powder; best self-made: I didn't find a better recipe in English but the following link shows one easy to follow:
www.youtube.com/watch?v=iDE0Y2hoYZE

The pancake also tastes delicious when you serve it with goat's cheese and spinach or with leeks, eggs, cream and sunflower seeds;

¼ bunch of parsley	chop and sprinkle a or coriander on the pancake filling

Sweets without remorse

Pineapple Kiwi Cream

1 fresh pineapple slice	peel, dice
2 kiwis	peel and mix with
2 tbsp sweet whey powder	and
½ - 1 tsp Spirulina	with a fork; spread
the cream on pineapple	cubes

Apricot bars

200 g dried apricots	and
150 g of dates or figs	soak in water
150 g raisins	wash and drain; add
1-2 tbsp Spirulina flour	and puree all the ingredients and the

soaking water in the blender; put the dough into a bowl and work

250 g ground almonds	into the mixture and spread the dough onto

a baking sheet covered with parchment paper; sprinkle with chufa sedge or coconut flakes. Depending on the weather you can let it dry in the sun or in the oven at 50°C by clamping a cooking spoon or towel in between to keep the door open. After 6 to 8 hours cut into large pieces; store them dry and airtight.

Banana cashew cake

2 ripe bananas puree with
4 tbsp of coconut oil,
2 tbsp erythritol/xylitol
1 pi sea salt and
1 handful cashew nuts in a blender; stir in
5 tbsp of coconut flour fill dough in a springform; go on as in
citrus cake; blend
2 ripe bananas with
1 tbsp of Spirulina flour; spread over the cake; sprinkle 1 handful cashew nuts over it

Fig sesame taler

6-8 fresh figs mix with
100 g sesame seeds,
1 tbsp Spirulina flour and
1 tsp baobab powder; form sm
balls, flatten

Lentil granola (gluten free)

1 cup of lentils mill; soak ½ hour
1 tbsp chia seeds in 5 tbsp water and mix
with the ground lentils; add
¼ TL sea salt
cinnamon or vanilla
cashews or almonds, germinated
pumpkin/pine or sunflower seeds
dried Fruits (figs, apples, cranberries)
honey or maple syrup and
3 tbsp coconut oil mix everything well; spread
on a baking sheet with baking paper and let it dry in the oven at 50°C with a towel tucked between the door until the desired crispiness is reached. Pour over almond or rice milk and sprinkle 1 tsp of Spirulina powder on it.

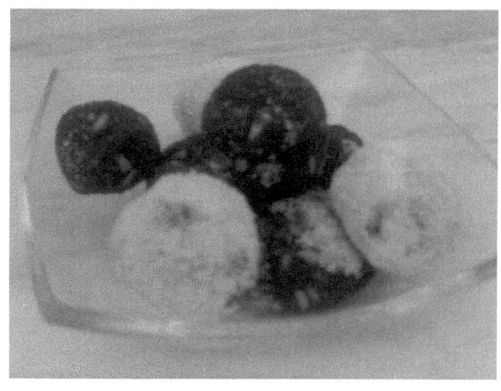

Nougat balls

6 tbsp chufa sedge flakes
1-2 tbsp carob powder
2 tsp Spirulina powder
1 tbsp coconut flour or
sweet whey powder stir until smooth with
3-4 tbsp coconut or hemp oil; sweeten w.
stevia or xylitol refine with
1 pi sea salt and some grated
organic lemon peel

Form balls, roll them in coconut chips and refrigerate. Instead of chufa sedge flakes, you can use chia seeds, soaked in ½ cup of water

Strawberry cake

4 tbsp of chia seeds soak in
¼ cup of water liquefy
¼ organic lemon
2 hf almonds
4 tbsp coconut oil
1 pi of sea salt and ½ of
the strawberries you can also use any sea-
sonal fruit mix
Erythritol or Stevia to sweeten; in a dish mix
6 tbsp. coconut flour
1 tbsp Spirulina flour
½ tsp bicarb and the rest of the fruits;
mix and add some more flour if the dough is too wet. fill it in a greased springform, decorate with fruits and coconut chips. In preheated oven bake at 90°C

for 1½ to 2 hours. For raw food quality 6 to 8 hours at 50°C by clamping a cooking spoon or towel in between to keep the door open.

Sweet carrot casserole

4-5 egg yolk	batter with
5 tbsp sesame oil	or walnut oil; add
1 tbsp Spirulina flour	
4 large carrots	grated
20-25 dates	chopped and
1 cup cooked millet	or
6-8 tbsp of flour	beat

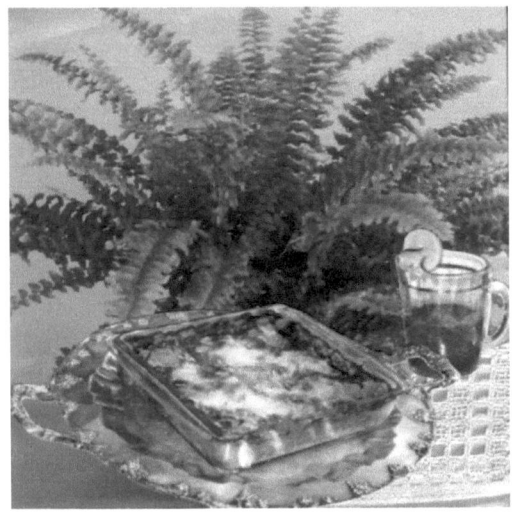

4-5 egg whites	until stiff; season with
stevia & cinnamon	or ginger or to choice

Bake in a greased gratin dish at 90°C for 2 hours in the oven. You can do the casserole also with hearty ingredients, e. g., with corn or bean sprouts; Season with herbal salt and cayenne.

Walnut balls

10 walnuts	milled
½ cup berries	or a grated apple mix with
1 tsp Spirulina powder	
1 pi stevia	and
1 tsp honey	or agave sirup

Form balls, roll into coconut flakes and decorate with two walnut halves each.

Walnut/almond plum bar

1 can of California plums	mix with
some water	in a blender; add
200 g walnuts	or
germinated almonds	coarsely ground &
4 tbsp goji berries	to the pulp, spread
2 tbsp Spirulina flour	over it and mix in

Spread the dough about ½ cm thick (0,2 inches) on a greased baking sheet or baking paper; dry at 50°C for a few hours; keep the door open with a spoon. The drying time depends on the degree of humidity. If you thicken with sweet whey powder you can shorten the time.

Citrus and almond cake

4 tbsp of chia seeds for 20 minutes soak in	
¼ cup of water	combine with
4 tbsp coconut flour	
1 hulled vanilla pod	mill in a coffee grinder
1 tbsp guar gum	and
1 pi of salt	in a bowl; liquefy
1 organic orange	peeled; divide into eighth remove cores
1 organic orange	unpeeled with

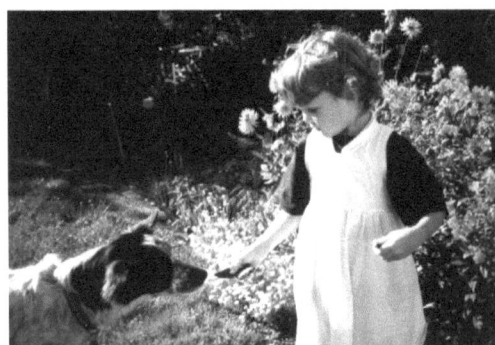

Katja lures Sandy with a delicious Spirulina fruit bar

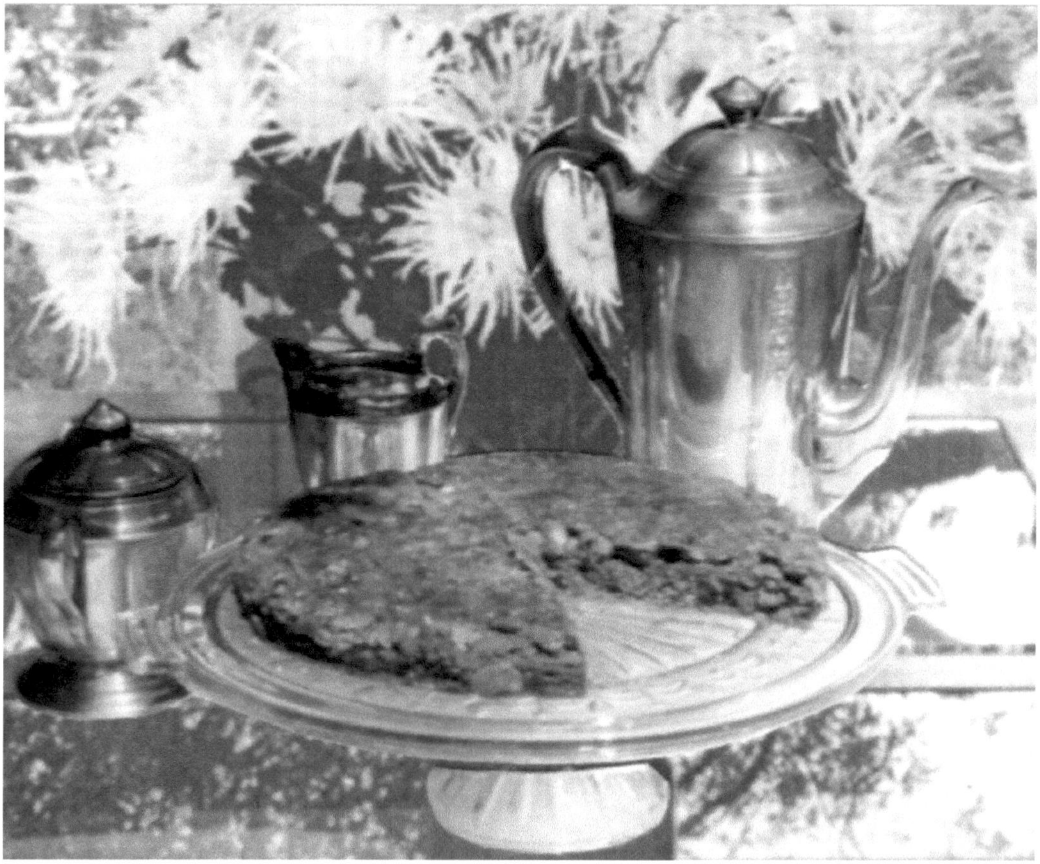

½ cup coconut milk or sweet cream,
1 tbsp erythritol or other sweeteners without calories
3 tbsp coconut oil and
1 cup almonds in a blender and put it in the bowl; peel
2 kiwifruit chop; add to the dough; fill it in
a greased springform, cover with orange and kiwi slices and decorate with coconut chips. Continue as on the Strawberry cake on page 83.

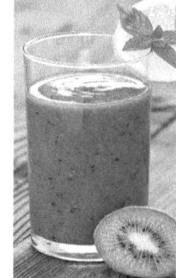

Beverages for body, mind and soul
Drinks for detoxification
Coriander and cucumber juice
½ bunch coriander (cilantro) liquefy with
1 tsp Spirulina flour
¼ tsp sea salt
2 tbsp olive oil and
1 pi cayenne in a blender

Wild herbs shake (brain and nerve food)
Liquefy a bundle of wild herbs, e. g., wild mint, borage, cuckoo flower, sorrel, willowherb, daisy, mallow, dandelion and other meadow offerings with 1 cup of water or carrot juice, 2 tbsp hemp or camelina oil, 1 tsp

Spirulina powder, 1 tbsp onion cubes and ¼ tsp sea, stone or crystal salt in a blender. Add some sunflower seeds or ½ avocado to get a creamy flavor. You can refine the shake with kiwi or lemon. The basket full of wild growing herbs on the photo on the left we collected far from exhaust gasses. Microorganisms live on the wild plants. They are good for digestion and the immune system. Also, because of the desensitizing effect of the wild herb blossom dust too thorough washing is not necessary with regard to the vitamin B12 synthesis.

Anti-aging goodies for losing weight

You can enjoy these superfoods for the arteries, brains, and skin like the Hollywood stars at Juliano's Planet Raw on Santa Monica Boulevard or at Erewhon Bio-Supermarket. But for each day the own kitchen is best. Perhaps you wonder why I use coconut oil or coconut flour in my creamy drinks and desserts against love handles and spare tires. Since one year, I'm using organic coconut oil for cooking, frying, baking, skin, and hair. Otherwise, nothing has changed in my diet and lifestyle. Still, I lost 3 kilos. If you want to learn and slim by experience, just try it.

The raw or native coconut oil is pressed in a gentle process that preserves the valuable ingredients leaving the beneficial fatty acids unchanged. It also includes monolaurin, the glycerol ester of lauric acid that destroys the outer envelope of unwanted bacteria, viruses, and fungi. This natural fatty acid also occurs in the mother's milk. In the body, it is effective against disease-causing viruses, bacteria, and fungi including fungal infections, herpes viruses, measles, flu and many other infectious diseases. Coconut oil also helps with chronic fatigue and digestive problems as well as with Alzheimer's, ADS, diabetes cancer and heart diseases.

Coconut kiwi shake

1 coconut   drill 2 holes; mix milk with
¼ fruit pulp
2 kiwis   with or without the peel
1 pi stevia or other sweeteners without calories
1 tbsp Spirulina flour and
1 piece of ginger   or ½ tsp powder
                  in a blender

If you do not want to lose weight, you can add half a cup of sweet or coconut cream.

Pineapple raspberry smoothie

1 slice of pineapple fresh, peeled; liquefy with
1 handful raspberries
½ cup coconut milk or apple juice and
1 tsp Spirulina flour in a blender; for a creamy
                  flavor add 1 tbsp coconut cream

Anti-inflammatory drinks

Fig baobab smoothie

4 fresh figs   or 1 banana mix with
2 kiwis
2 tsp baobab powder *)
2 tsp of rose hip powder *)
1 tsp Spirulina powder
1 piece of ginger   and
¼ l almond milk   (mix 1 handful of almonds in 1 cup of water)

*) www.detoxtrading.co.uk/rosehip-powder.htm
www.goldener-zweig.de

Cherry papaya smoothie

1 cup of cherries   mix in a blender with
½ papaya incl. 15 seeds and
2 tbsp sunflower seeds germinated

Spinach apple smoothie

1 handful spinach leaves mix with 8 pieces of
1 apple, unpeeled   seeds removed
1 avocado pulp

1 tbsp of hemp oil or pumpkin seeds
½ tsp turmeric
1 piece of ginger or ½ tsp powder and
½ liter of pure water or green tea
in a blender; season with salt and pepper and / or vegetable broth powder

Liquid soul comforter

Banana apple shake

2 bananas — peel, cut into pieces
1 unpeeled sweet apple — cut roughly
3 figs or 5 dates — and
1 tbsp Spirulina powder — mix with
2 cups of spring water — in a blender

This brain food ensures regular bowel movements and mental health. It strengthens the bones and nerves.

B vitamin shake

3 tbsp flaxseed — mill finely or
1 handful almonds — germinated; mix with
½ l rice milk
2 tbsp sweet whey powder and
2 tsp Spirulina flour — in a blender
allow to swell for 5 min

Chocolate smoothie

1 tbsp cocoa beans — soak ½ h with
1 tbsp chia seeds — in 100 ml of water in a blender; mix along with
2 apple quarters
1 piece of ginger
1 tbsp erythritol
1 tbsp coconut oil — and
1 tsp Spirulina flour

Instead of cocoa beans, you can also use cocoa or carob powder.

Drinks for guts and guns

Avocado apple drink

1 small avocado — mix the pulp with
1 acid apple — cut in 8 pieces
½ diced papaya — or pineapple
1 tsp Spirulina powder — and
1 cup grapefruit juice — in a blender; add
½ teaspoon fennel
or anise powder — to taste

Cucumber shake

½ cucumber — brush, cut in cubes liquefy along with
3 tbsp of sweet cream — a little water and
2 tsp Spirulina flour — season with
sea salt and mustard — trim with

1 tablespoon parsley, finely chopped and
2 tbsp chopped dill

Blueberry smoothy

100 g blueberries — mix together with
5 dates or figs (optional)
1 tsp Spirulina — and
1 cup of water — in a blender; add
1 pi sea salt or stone salt — and refine with
¼ grated organic lemon

Red currant sorbet

100 g currants — liquefy with
2 to 3 ice cubes
1 tsp Spirulina powder
1 cup of water — and
1 pi stevia — in a blender
for a creamier taste add
3 tbsp sunflower seeds — soaked for 6 hours
1 pi salt & chili — to taste

Keep every sip in your mouth for a few seconds. Thus the active ingredients of Spirulina can enter the bloodstream through the oral mucosa. The preheating promotes the production of stomach acid.

Recent studies on vitamin B12 analogs are bad news, especially for vegans and vegetarians. However, other studies conclude that algae can raise vitamin B12 serum levels. Because Vitamin B12 deficiency can be undetected for many years, to be sure we better avoid eating vitamin B12 sources together with Spirulina or take vitamin B12 in the form of drops, best as methylcobalamin. Because it is directly usable by the body and does not have to be converted like cyanocobalamin. I give me every 3 months vitamin B12 injections in the form of hydroxocobalamin as it has a good depot effect meaning it has a prolonged release period and therefore a longer effect. The liver can store approximately 2000-5000 µg of vitamin B12. Because the body needs only 3.0 µg per day, emptying takes several years.

If recipes require eggs, you can replace them with soaked or ground or soaked chia or linseed, carob gum or bananas. Instead of cream, you can use coconut or soy cream.

Conclusion

"You see things; and you say, 'Why?' But I dream things that never were; and I say, 'Why not?'"

George Bernard Shaw

If I have succeeded in showing you how little we need to stay healthy, I'd be delighted. However, whether or not you will steer clear of hospitals and doctors' offices, is your decision. Not everyone feels as a Kamikaze Cowboy, such as Dirk Benedikt (1991). At age 27, the A-team actor could cure his prostate cancer only with strict macrobiotic diet. Still, it would be beneficial if you could regularly consume Spirulina to protect your body and the environment. We do not have to deal with a lot of different medicines since the algae harmonize the whole organism. They protect not only us but also our plants, the earth, and the water, which Viktor Schauberger called the blood of the earth. If we use fewer chemicals for pest control and chemical drugs, we ensure better drinking water. Since a Wiesbaden symposium of drugs in waters in 1998, we know that sewage treatment plants are not able to eliminate urine excreted drugs during reprocessing. The graduate engineer Thomas Junker from the Odenwald had built an award-winning miniature sewage plant. He studied a radioactive marked antibiotic substance in the laboratory for biodegradability. The researcher ´still detected almost 93% of the drug. Most antibiotics would, therefore, enter the rivers! (Meyer 2015)

With chemicals, pesticides, petroleum and radioactive pollution we ruin us and our planet. The marine pollution with plastic and the disaster in Japan show this terribly clearly. Thus we better claim free energy as described in my book HOW WATER CONNECTS OUR WORLDS and bioplastic from algae as produced by Algopack (see p. 34).

Tesla's space energy converters based on the phenomenon of rotating energy fields could have moved vehicles and illuminate houses for about 100 years. The commercialization was prevented by a selfish banker. Due to declining resources, we are more concerned with the issue of free energy.

Let's not allow ourselves to demur on acting by the phrase "We can not turn the wheel back". Let's jump from the cart before the wheel breaks! If we let our energies flow into sustainable projects, we serve the protection of life. With a large-scale breeding of Spirulina and the conversion to the new techniques in the energy industry, hunger and unemployment could be eliminated worldwide in a few years. See my book *HOW WATER CONNECTS OUR WORLDS*, chapter "Free energy for free people.

We create our reality with our thoughts. Donald Neale Walsch's words help make it a heaven on earth. All that happens is the external physical manifestation of our innermost thoughts, ideas, and decisions about who we are and who we choose to be.

> *Condemn not, therefore, those aspects of life which you disagree. Seek instead to change them, and the conditions that made them possible.*
>
> *Behold the darkness, yet curse it not. Rather, be a light unto the darkness, and so transform it. Let your light so shine before men, that those who stand in the darkness will be illuminated by the light of your being, and all of you will see, at last, Who You really Are.*
>
> *Be a Bringer of the Light. For your light can do more than illuminate your own path. Your light can be the light which truly lights the world.*
>
> *The world waits for you. Heal it. Now. In the place where you are. There is much you can do.* (Walsch 1999, page 96).

We can protect ourselves from all adversities by listening to our inner voice, whether it represents ourselves, deceased relatives, or a higher intelligence. Let's create our own knowledge through attention in our daily lives by not ignoring and repressing synchronicities but integrating these so-called coincidences into our routine and learning from them. Then we no longer need to believe because we feel spiritual helpers that always surround us. It is also my experience that led me to realize that the water is an interface between the physical and metaphysical reality. In my above-mentioned book and in my blog reports I have shown this: www.marianne-e-meyer.com

If we consume the light food regularly, we get into a higher vibration and perceive spiritual messages. By eating light food and drinking water or activated water, we also serve our environment and health. When we use Spirulina as a dietary supplement thousands of people are less suffering from iatrogenic diseases which are caused by the doctor. The examples of drugs taken from the market heat up the debate repeatedly whether synthetic drugs are tested sufficiently. This points to the following:

It exceeds physician's skills to examine all side effects of medications as there are far too many.

Diseases caused by doctors include candida yeast infections after antibiotics if a destroyed intestinal flora is not rebuilt. Also vaccination complications (according to Dr. med. Gerhard Buchwald: Vaccination: A Business based on Fear) after influenza inoculations, but above all after the MMR (measles, mumps, and rubella) vaccine which is associated with autism and intestinal disease and after vaccinations against whooping cough.

After three years of testing with the Apnea Breathing Monitor for SIDS (Sudden Infant Death Syndrome), Dr. Viera Schreibner announced that vaccinations against whooping cough slow down breathing such as sometimes death occurs (Simon Jones, "A shot in the dark." Investigate April/May 2001). As pathologists are never investigating vaccine complications in autopsies of sudden childhood death, it can be assumed that the SIDS shortly after the immunization of the child is caused mostly by reactions of the vaccine. Parents convinced by the immunization theory or dogmatic medicine better add some Spirulina powder to the baby's diet a few days before and after vaccinations. Perhaps this could lessen vaccination ills as discovered by Julena Meroti of the National Advisory Group on Autopsy Inc. in New Zealand. At her request whether the vaccines ever had been tested on humans, the Ministry of Health told the tests were carried out overseas. But US doctors disproved this claim. The famous pediatrician Dr. Robert Mendelsohn said:

> "There has never been a single vaccine in this country that has ever been submitted to a controlled scientific study. They never took a group of 100 people who were candidates for a vaccine, gave 50 of them a vaccine and left the other 50 alone, and measured the outcome. And since that has never been done, that means if you want to be kind, you will call vaccines an unproven remedy. If you want to be accurate, you'll call the people who give vaccines quacks."

See also: http://rawfed.com/vax/50things.html

Many Africans believe they have been given AIDS by mass vaccination as men and women are equally affected in Africa. In industrialized countries, homosexual and drug-dependent men account for 80 % of persons with AIDS. In Africa, women and men are equally affected. The reason is that women and children are used for any dirty work without protective masks, e. g., they work with pesticides we prohibit. Also, women are genital-mutilated in many places. At each birth, the wound suture must be opened again and sewn again. This weakening of the immune system the algae can prevent. If they first perceive their effect themselves, they can keep the doctor at bay.

Acknowledgments

Last, but certainly not least, I'd like to thank the people who have contributed to the improvement of the book: Prof. Peter H. Duesberg, Dr. Stefan Lanka, Stephan Kuhl and Dr. med. Dirk-Bijan Zarrinnam for tips and reviews.

I am grateful to Prof. Günter Kahl for information about his specialty enzymes, the company Cyanotech and Marcus Rohrer for information, photos and reports, Dr. Amha Belay from Earthrise for information and photos, the companies Dr. Hittich, Spira Verde, Sanatur and Pure Planet for articles and photos, Halima Neumann for information and help with recipes, Jürgen Görke for Kirlian photographs, C.-P. Meyer for formulation assistance.

Also, my heartfelt thanks for the valuable contributions that many others have made by providing ideas and experience reports.

Though I list the following persons jointly, I am aware of the individual contribution: Barbara Simonsohn, Renate Kaiser-Alexnat, Erwin Albe, J. P. Jourdan, Heide Bayer, Ursula and Werner Keim, B. and H. Sommer, Susanne Würtz, Hildegard Assmus, W. and M. Rohde, Sylvia Priewe, Renate Janzen, Evelyn and Elisabeth Fleischer, Marianne Müller, Anneliese Umbreit, Alwine Holschuh, and all the souls related to me or connected with me for spiritual help.

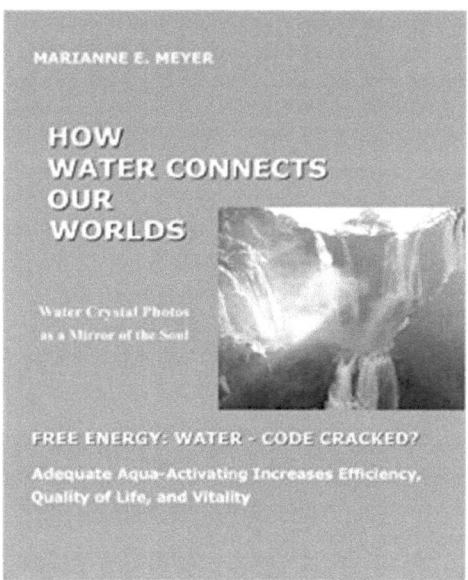

This captivating book wins by a clear statement on the mystery of changeability and storage ability of the water. Inge Schneider, head of the Swiss Jupiter-Verlag, found in her book review in the NET-Journal the author's findings that the water is the "interface between the physical and metaphysical reality" particularly appealing.

The reader will find disturbing facts about the quality of commercial waters. Anyone who believes that a tap water is clean, is encouraged to think and act. M. Meyer advises to activating water adequately. After all, who tastes for the first time naturally vitalized, oxygenated and alkaline water from the tap, want to drink no more soda water from plastic bottles. Pure water is the ideal solution for all health problems, especially if they affect the brain.

Ultimately, the author introduces free energy researchers and their technologies. She also shows what to do, so space energy can soon flow in all households.

ISBN 978-3734736919 104 p. 17x22cm €7,99

Bibliography

Abdel-Daim, MM et al.: Anti-inflammatory and imunomodulatory effects of Spirulina platensis in comparison to Dunaliella salina in acetic acid-induced rat experimental colitis. Immunopharmacol Immunotixol. 2015 Apr;37(2): 126-39

Balch, JF, Balch, PH: Prescription for Nutritional Healing, Garden City Park, New York,1997

Banji, D et al.: Investigation on the role of Spirulina platensis in ameliorating behavioural changes, thyroid dysfunction and oxidative stress in offspring of pregnant rats exposed to fluoride. Food Chem. 2013 Sep 1;140 (1-2) 321-31

Batmanghelidj, Faridum: Wasser, die gesunde Lö-Lösung. Freiburg 1997

Becker, EW, Jakover, B, Luft, D, Schmülling, RM: Clinical and biochemical evaluations of the alga Spirulina with regard to its application in the treatment of obesity: a double-blind cross-over study. Nutr. Rep. Int. 33 (1986) 565-74

Benedikt, Dirk: Mein Leben als Kamikaze Cowbboy, Holthausen 1991

Benner, K U: Gesundheit und Medizin heute. Augsburg 1994

Bermejo-Bescós P et al.: Neuroprotection by Spirulina platensis protean extract and phycocyanin against iron-induced toxicity in SH-SY5Y neuroblastoma cells.Toxicol In Vitro. 2008; Sep;22 (6) 1496-502

Bragg, Paul C und Patricia: Wasser. Das größte Gesundheitsgeheimnis. Die schockierende Wahrheit über Wasser, Ritterhude, 4. Aufl. 1992

Challem, Jack. J, Spirulina: What it is ... the health benefits it can give you, Good Health Guide Series, Keats Publishing Inc. New Canaan Connecticut,1981

Buser K et al.: Krankheit und soziale Lage, Sonderfall Neurodermitis, Gesundheitswesen. 1989

Chen T, Wong YS: In vitro antioxidant and antiproliferative activities of selenium-containing phycocyanin from selenium-enriched Spirulina platensis. J Agric Food Chem 2008 Jun 25;56 (12):4352-8

Cingi, C et al.: The effects of spirulina on allergic rhinitis. Eur Arch Otorhinolaryngol. 2008 Oct; 265 (10) 1219-23

Clement, G et al: (inventors; Institute Francais de Petrol, assignee). Wound treating medicaments containing algae. Fr. M. 5279 (Int. Cl. A61k), 11 Sep. 1967.

Collier, Renate: Wie neugeboren durch Darmreinigung. München 1995

Devi, MA, Venkataraman, L.V.: Hypocholesterolemic effect of bluegreen algae Spirulina platensis in albino rats. Nutr Rep Int 28 (1983) 519-30

Fukino, H, Takagi, Y, Yamane, Y.: Effect of Spirulina (S. platensis) on the renal toxicity induced by inorganic mercury and cisplatin. Eisei Kagaku, 36 (1990) 5

Galmén, K, Höjer, J: Iron intoxication-poisoning with easily accessible medicines. Lakartidningen 2014 Sep 17-23

Gershwin, ME, Belay, A: Spirulina in human nutrition and health. Journal of Applied Psychology 21(6):747-748 · December 2009

Gruben, Rozalind: Vegetarierkonkress Widnau, CH 1999

Gupta, S et al.: Spirulina protects against rosiglitazone induced osteoporosis in insulin resistance rats. Diabetes Res Clin Pract.2010 Jan;87(1)38-43

Gutiérrez-Rebolledo, GA et al.: Antioxidant Effect of Spirulina (Arthrospira) maxima on Chronic I flammation Induced by Freund's Complete Adj vant in Rats. 2015 Aug;18(8):865-71

Hayashi, O et al.: Enhancement of antibody production in mice by dietary Spirulina platensis. J. Nutr.Sci. Vitaminol (Tokyo) 40-5 (1994) 431-41

Hayashi, T et al.: Calcium spirulan, an inhibitor of enveloped virus replication, from a blue-green alga Spirulina platensis. J.Nat.Prod. 59-1 (1996) 83-7

Hayashi, T.: Studies on evaluation of natural products for antiviral effects and their applications Yakugaku Zasshi. 2008 Jan;128(1) 61-79

Helmke-Hausen, Monika: Die Botschaft der Früchte, Freiburg 1998

Hoffmann, Peter (Hrsg.): Positivlisten Lebensmittel, Frankfurt 1995

Huang ZX et al.: Protective effects of polysaccharide of Spirulina platensis and Sargassum thunbeergii on vascular of alloxan induced diabetic rats. Zhongguo Zhong Yao Za Zhi. 2005 Feb;30 (3) 211-5

Huang, Z, Zheng, W: Antagonistic effects of Se-rich Spirulina platensis on rat liver fibrosis. Wei Sheng Yan Jiu. 2007 Jan; 36 (1) 34-6 17424844

Ichimura M et al.: Phycocyanin prevents hyper tension and low serum adiponectin level in a rat model of metabolic syndrome. Nutr Res. 2013 May;33(5) 397-405

Iwata K et al.: Effects of Spirulina platensis on plasma lipoprotein lipase activity in fructose-induced hyperlipidemic rats. J Nutr Sci Vitaminol. 1990 Apr;36 (2) 165-71

Jorjani, G, Amirani, P: Antibacterial activities of spirulina platensis. Maj. limy Puz. Danisk. Jundi Shap, 1 (1978) 14-18

Kato, T, Takemoto, K: Effects of Spirulina on hypercholesterolemia and fatty liver in rats. Saitama Med. College, Japan. Japan Nutr foods Assoc. Jour. 1984, 37:321

Katz M et al.: A compound herbal preparation (CHP) in the treatment of children with ADHD: a randomized controlled trial. J Atten Disord. 2010 Nov;14(3):281-91

Kawanishi, Y et al: Regulatory effects of Spirulina complex polysaccharides on growth of murine RSV-M glioma cells through Toll-like receptor 4.Microbiol Immunol 2013 Jan;57 (1) 63-73

Kim, HM et al.: Inhibitory effect of mast cell mediated immediate-type allergic reactions in rats by Spirulina. Biochem.Pharmacol. Apr. 1; 55 -7 (1998) 1071-6

Kim LS et al.: Efficacy of methylsulfonylmethane (MSM) in osteoarthritis pain of the knee: a pilot clinical trial. Osteoarthritis Cartilage. 2006 Mar; 14(3):286-94

Kim, NH et al.: The effect of hydrolyzed Spirulina by malted barley on forced swimming test in ICR mice. Int J Neurosci 2008 Nov; 118(11): 1523-33

Köhler, Barbara et al.: Photonenemission. Eine neue Methode zur Erfassung der Qualität! Von Lebensmitteln. Deutsche Lebensmittel-Rund schau, Jg. 87, 3 (1991) 78-83

Koníčková R et al.: Anti-cancer effects of bluegreen alga Spirulina platensis, a natural source of bilirubin-like tetrapyrrolic compounds. Ann Hepatol 2014 Mar-Apr;13 (2) 273-83

Kugler, H et al.: Life Extenders and Memory Boosters. Health Quest Publication, Reno 1994

Kulshreshtha, A et al.: Spirulina in health care management. Curr Pharm Biotechnol 2008 Oct; 9 (5): 400-5

Kumari, RP et al.: C-phycocyanin modulates selenite-induced cataractogenesis in rats. Biol Trace Elem Res. 2013 Jan;151 (1) 59-67

Li B et al.: Effects of CD59 on antitumoral activities of phycocyanin from Spirulina platensis. Biomed Pharmacother. 2005 Dec;59(10):551-60

Lobner M et al.: Enhancement of human adaptive immune responses by administration of a high-molecular-weight polysaccharide extract from the cyanobacterium Arthrospira platensis. J Med Food. 2008 Jun;11 (2) 313-22

Loseva, LP, Jurinok, HW: Ausleitung von Schwermetallen (Blei) mit der Mikroalge Spirulina platensis. In: Naturheilpraxis 05/2000

Lu, HK et al.: Preventive effects of Spirulina platensis on skeletal muscle damage under exercise-induced oxidative stress. Eur J Appl Physiol. 2006 Sep; 98 (2) 220-6. Epub 2006 Aug 30

Ma, QY et al.: Optimised extraction of β-carotene, from Spirulina platensis and hypoglycaemic effect in streptozotocin-induced diabetic mice. J Sci Food Agric. 2016 Mar 30;96(5):1783-9

Martinez-Nadal, NG: Antimicrobal activity of Spirulina. Paper presented at X International of Microbiology, Mexico City, Aug. 1970

Maruta T et al.: Optimists vs. pessimists: survival rate among medical patients over a 30 year period. Mayo Clinic Proc. 75 (2000) 140-3

Majdoub, H: Anticoagulant activity of a sulfated polysaccharide from the green alga Arthrospira platensis. Biochem Biophys Acta 2009 Oct; 1790(10):1377-81

Mao, T K et al.: Effects of a Spirulina-based dietary supplement on cytokine production from allergic rhinitis patients. J Med Food. 2005 Spring; 8 (1) 27-30

Marin-Prida J et al: Phycocyanobilin promotes PC12 cell survival and modulates immune and inflammatory genes and oxidative stress markers in acute cerebral hypoperfusion in rats. Toxicol Appl Pharmacol 2013 June 2.

Mathew, B: Sankaranarayanan, R. et al. Evaluation of chemoprevention of oral cancer with Spirulina fusiform. Nutr Cancer 24 -2 (1995) 197-202

Meyer, Marianne Erika.: Spirulina, das blaugrüne Wunder. Aitrang 7. Auflage 2006

Wasser verbindet die Welten, Norderstedt 2016

Müller-Wohlfahrt, Hans-Wilhelm: So schützen Sie Ihre Gesundheit. München 2000

Nakaya, N, Honma, Y, Goto, Y: Cholesterol lowering effect of Spirulina Nutr. Rep. Int. 37 (1988) 1329-37.

Neumann, Halima: Stop Krebs, MS, AIDS Grüne Lebenselixiere. Spiraverde.de

Ou, Y et al.: Antidiabetic potential of phycocyanin: effects on KKAy mice. Pharm Biol. 2013 May;51 (5) 539-44

Pane, L et al.: Effect of extracts from Spirulina platensis bioaccumulating cadmium and zinc on L929 cells. Ecotox Envir Saf.2008May;70 (1) 121-6. Epub 2007 Jul 26

Passwater, Richard. The New Supernutrition, Pocket Books, New York 1991

Peschanel, Mathias: Isolierung und Charakterisierung pharmakologisch relevanter Verbindungen aus der Alge *Spirulina platensis.* Universität Kiel, 1996 (ISBN-3-9804010-5-7)

Popp, Fritz-Albert.: Biophotonen-Analyse der Lebensmittelqualität. In: Meier-Ploeger, A, Vogtmann. H (Hrsg.): Lebensmittelqualität (1988) Die Botschaft der Nahrung. Fischer alternativ, Frankfurt 1993

Qureshi, M A et al.: Immunomodulary effect of Spirulina supplementation in chickens. North Carolina State. Pub. in Proc. of 44th Western Poultry Disease Conference, 1995, 117-20.

Roy, KR et al. Alteration of mitochondrial membrane popotential by Spirulina platensis C-phycocyanin induces apoptosis in the doxorubicinresistant human hehepatocellular-carcinlichtenergieoma cell line HepG2 Biotechnol Appl Biochem. 2007 Jul;47 (Pt 3) 159-67

Saini MK, Sanyal SN: Piroxicam and c-phycocyanin prevent colon carcinogenesis by inhibition of membrane fluidity and canonical Wnt/β-catenin signaling while up-regulating ligand dependent transcription factor PPARγ. Biomed Pharmacother. 2014 Jun;68(5):537-50.

Santillan, C.: Cultivation of Spirulina for human

consumption and for animal feed. International Congress of Food, Science and Technology. Madrid, September 1974

Seshadri C V: Large scale nutritional supplementation with Spirulin alga. All India Coordinates Project on Spirulina. Shri Amm Murugappa Chettiar Research Center (MCRC), Madras, India 1993

Shklar G, Schwartz J: Tumor necrosis factor in experimental cancer regression with alphatocopherol, beta-carotene, canthaxanthin and algae extract. Eur J Cancer Clin Oncol. 1988 May;24 (5) 839-50

Saini MK, Sanyal SN: Piroxicam and c-phycocyanin prevent colon carcinogenesis by inhibition of membrane fluidity and canonical Wnt/β-catenin signaling while up-regulating. Biomed Pharmacother. 2014 Mar 19

Selmi, C et al.: The effects of Spirulina on anemia and immune function in senior citizens. Cell Mol Immunol . 2011 May ;8(3)::248-54.

Simonsohn, Barbara. Stevia, sündhaft süß und urgesund. Oberstdorf 2010
Die Heilkraft der AFA-Alge. München 2000

Takai, Y, Hosoyamada, Y, Kato, T: Effect of water-soluble and water in soluble fractions of Spirulina over serum lipids and glucose resistance of rats. J. Jap. Soc. Nutr Food Sci. 44 (1991) 273-77

Takemoto, K: Iron transfer from spirulina to blood in rats. Saitama Med. Col., Japan, 1982, 62.

Takeuchi, T: Clinical experiences of administration of spirulina to patients with hypochr. Anemia Tokyo Medical and Dental Univ., Japan, 1978

Taniguchi, Masaharu: Leben aus dem Geiste. Freiburg 1994

Teas, J, Irhimeh, MR: Dietary algae and HIV/AIDS: proof of concept clinical data. J Appl Phycol. 2012 Jun;24 (3) 575-582

Tominaga, A et al.: Autonomous cure of damaged human intestinal epithelial cells by TLR2 and TLR4-dependent production of IL-22 in response to Spirulina polysaccharides. Int Immunophamacol. 2013 Dec;17(4):1009-19.

Upasani, CD, Balaraman R.: Protective effects of Spirulina on lead induced deleterious changes in the lipid peroxidation and endogenous antioxidants in rats. Phytotherapy Res. 17;4 (2003) 330-334

Vadiraja, BB et al.: Hepatoprotective effects of C-phycocyanin. Biochem. Biophys. Res. Commun. 19; 249 (1998) 428-31

Walsch, Neale Donald: Gespräche Mit Gott. Band 1-3, München 1997-99

Winter, FS et al.: The effect of Arthrospira platensis capsules on CD4 T-cells and anti-oxiatative capacity in a randomized pilot study of adult women infected with human immunodeiciency virus not under HAART in Yaoundé, Cameroon. Nutrients Jul 2014 23;6(7):2973-86

Yamada, K et al.: Bioavailability of dried asakusanori (porphyra tenera) as a source of Cobalamin (Vitamin B_{12}). Int J Vitam Nutr Res. 1999 Nov; 69 (6) 412-8

Yang, L et al.: Inhibitory effects of polysaccharide extract from Spirulina platensis on corneal neovascularization. Mol Vis. 2009 Sep 24;15:1951-61

Yogianti, F et al.: Inhibitory Effects of Dietary Spirulina platensis on UVB-Induced Skin Inflammatory Responses and Carcinogenesis. J Invest Dermatol. 2014 Apr 14. doi: 10.1038/jid.2014.188

Yoshinari, O et al.: Hepatoprotective effect of germanium-containing Spirulina in rats with d-galactosamine- and lipopolysaccharide-induced hepatitis. The British journal of nutrition (impact Factor: 3.45). 06/2013

Yuan X et al.: Impact of ammonia concentration on Spirulina platensis growth in an airlift photobioreactor. Bioresource techn., Febr. 2011, vol./is. 102/3 (3234-9), 1873-2976

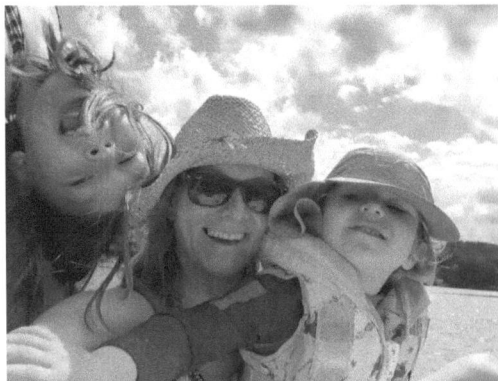

Susanne and her family takes Hawaiian Spirulina since 16 years

Index

Acne 9,76
Age spots 9,45,68,72
AIDS 9,18,19,44,47,51-55,73,76,93
Allergy 9,10,15,27,44,49,52,53,64,66,69,72,76,
Anemia 15,18,4142,46,47,54,56,57,62,69,72,76
Antibiotics 8,9,20,23,53,56,59,60,92,93
Aphtha 15
Arthritis 10,41,47,55,59,75,76,81,81,90
Astaxanthin 58
Autoimmune disease 14,72
Beta-carotene 14,42,49,58,61,68
Blood pressure 9,23,28,36,43,47,50,51,57,59,75
Calcium 7,16,17,24,25,43,46,50,52,65
Callus 9,57,72
Cancer 10,12,14-17,26,27,38-42,44,45,47-49,
    54,55,60,61,62,73-78,82,90,92
Cardiovascular diseases 25,42,43,46,47,49
Carotenoids 7,15,17,30,42,58
Cataract/Glaucoma 8,25,58,64
Chemical medicines 10,12,14,16,19,22,44,48,50
    52-54,60-62,66,71,73,78
Cholesterol 19,43,47,57,59,76
Colds 9,37,75
Colon cleansing 8,10,27,37,49,70
Concentration/lack of 28,60,75
Copper 7,14,28,40,47,68
Corticosteroids/cortisone 45,57,78
Cranberrys 13,37,71,86
Depression/melancholia 10,21,23,24,27,36,41
    45,48,52,59,60,68,76
Diabetes 10,14,15,17,25,36,43,50,51,64,76,90
Diet 11,12,16-20,22-29,31,36,38,40,45,48,50,
    62,63,69-71,76,82,89,92,93
Eye problems 8,10,25,36,42,45,58,64
Fat/body fat 9,13,16,26,28,40,43,45,47,48,50,
    57,60,62,71,78,90
Folic Acid 7,16,17,28,46,56,62,66
Forgetfulness 36,74
Free radicals 13,14,24,48
Fungi/yeast/parasites 7,22,31,56,71,72,76,90
Gamma-linolenic acid 7,10,15,43,50,57
Gastrointestinal 8,9,14,17,24-27,36,42,43,45,
    46,49,50,57,58,62,70,72,76,93

Goiter 72,75
Hashimoto 14
Hay, Louise, 9,54
Heavy metals 7,13,20,24,25,40,42,51,60,66
Herpes/cold sore 9,15,43,55,56,772,6,78,90,
Hot flashes 73
Immune deficiency 18,19,22,44,54,57
Impotence 74
Itching 52,53,72,74
Inflammation 16,25,41,43,46,50,51,57,58,60,
    62,67,74,76
Influenza/flu 9,56,90,93
Kidney problems 12,13,24,25,28,39,40,62-64,75
Liver/gallbladder 8,10,12,13,24-28,39,44-50,
    57,61-63,76,78,91
Magnesium 7,16,17,24,26-28,31,39,42,47,52,60
Manganese 7,14,18,40,41,48,50,68
Mood Fluctuation 15,23,66,67
MS (multiple sclerosis) 14,21,51,52,55
Neurodermatitis/eczema 24,43,51,72,76
Niacin (vitamin B3) 7,18,24,45,71
Night blindness 15,45,58
Osteoporosis 43,46,47,76
Pain 9,16,23,28,36,45,46,49,54,57,58,62,67,69,
    72,74-78
Parkinson 16,17,21,49,51,52
Penicillin 61.66,67,93
Pesticides 7,9,11,16,17,41,42,46,51,55,60,66,
    92,94
Phenylalanine 7,24,28,60,67
Photosynthesis 9,32
Pregnancy 19,53,56,64,65
Prevention 12-17,19,21,24,25,33,38-48,50-58,71,
    75,77,92,94
Psyllium husk 2.8,27,71,83,85
Radioactive Substances 10,13,17,18,20,25,31,
    40,60,63,64,78,92
Reiki 9,53
Retinal hemorrhage 58
Rheumatoid 14,28,49,55,57,59,74,76
Sarcoidosis 76
Selenium 7,14,16,34,39,48,63,68,
Sulfonamides 57,78

Superoxide dismutase (SOD) 7,10,14,15,24,40,
41,50,57,67,68
Tryptophan 7,24,45,60,67
Valine 7, 67
Vitamin B5 (pantothenic acid) 7,16,45
Vitamin B12 7,21,24,36,41,42,45,46,56,66,67,
89,91
Vitamin B12 analogs 21,36,42
Vitamin B12 deficiency 41,91
Vitamin E 7,14,16,17,45,48,50,56,62,68
Warts 15,76

Since I do not find any handbook on the Cranberry in English, my next project after *Family Code* will be to translate mine. So, for the Cranberry season 2017, you can be well informed about the health-promoting power berry.

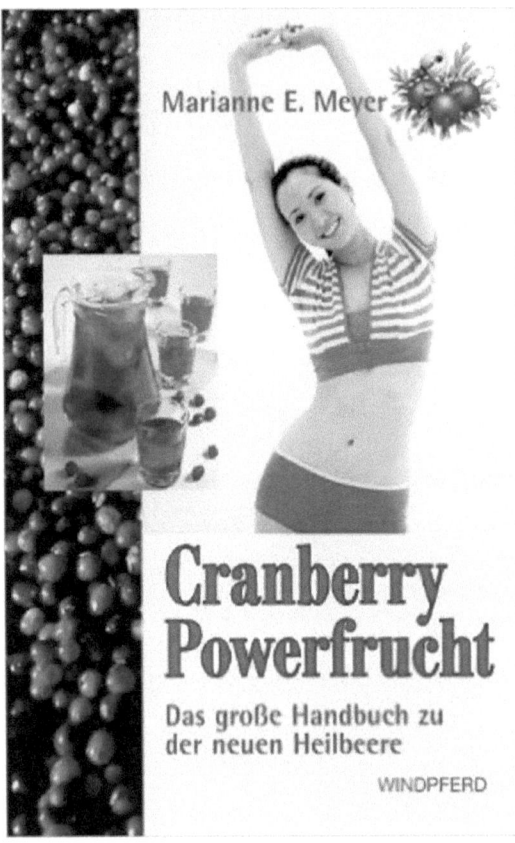

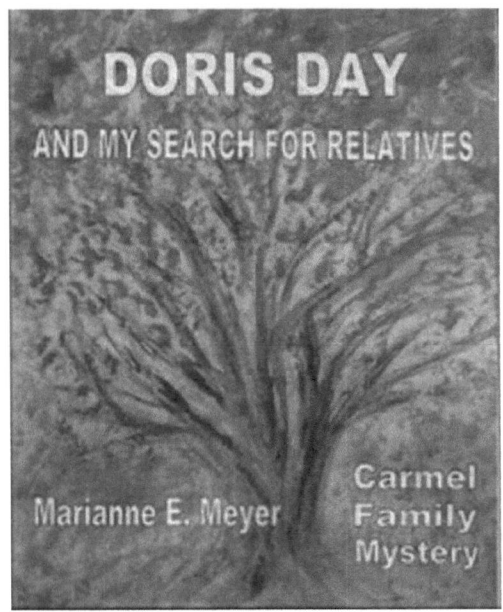

In this captivating spiritual novel, you take part in Marianne's exciting life on four continents realizing that we are all interconnected, and families have their value system for generations. This code of own rules, sayings and communication styles is also working when the family members live on different continents without knowing each other.

The book represents a bridge connecting the land of the living and the land of the dead. It shows that there is neither guilt nor chance or luck but only cause and effect that can be poles apart for many centuries and incarnations. Happiness, bad luck, and coincidence are only concepts for the unrecognized law. And who does not learn suffers. The only thing that remains which connects the worlds, the only meaning of life is LOVE.

Shortly, there will be a new revised edition of this book with the title *FAMILY CODE* for €9,99 (ISBN 978-3741282331). There will be no colored photos as in this version.

ISBN 978-3735792822 188 p. 17x22 cm €12,90

In the summer of 1995, I visited with a friend, the three freeway hours southeast of L. A. located Spirulina producer Earthrise Farms in the preparation of my doctoral thesis *Studies conducted on persons with immune deficiency diseases who used the food supplement Spirulina to enhance their immune system.* Next an excerpt from *Family Code,* the new edition of the book on the left since it shows in short the history and production of Spirulina:

"We had cut through the dry flickering heat of the Californian desert until the algae odor made us stop. Watching the dark blue-green iridescent surface in the huge ponds felt like visiting a church. Instead of marveling the Madonna, we watched the growth of ascendants of the very cyanobacteria that some 4½ billion years ago created the oxygen atmosphere. This first photosynthetic life form split water molecules with the help of sunlight thereby making their own food from surrounding gasses and minerals. From CO_2 they synthesized carbohydrates, from nitrogen via the amino acids protein. Thus they transformed Earth into a life-friendly system.

Had they also been the manna the Israelis had been fed on in the desert? Had the chosen ones been victims of an ET experiment? The 40-year duration and the intact clothes and sandals would account for this theory, so the stolen gold: the lifted offer for God.

In the southern California desert, a blazing heat of 43 degrees Celsius prevailed. After we had signed a confirmation not to make photos and to use our observance for business reasons, we had the opportunity to keep an eye on the culture. The trichomes, the chief chemist Dr. Belay had us look at under the microscope, were all tightly spirally coiled as screws tapering towards both ends. He also showed us the culture in the big glass bottles and the bottles with the liquid minerals and trace minerals.

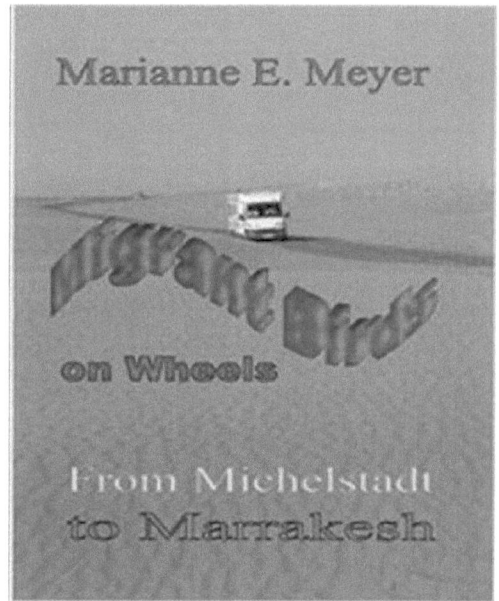

If your attention span suffers from this reading or you find health books difficult, I have an exciting book for you. Instead of getting the bullet directly through the eye, so to speak, I shoot from the back through the chest in the eye. Because in this novel, health tips come at best from medical miracles on two legs, which we have met in Morocco. In addition to Spirulina, there are other ways to get rid of blood and lung cancer or other modern epidemics.

Also, wintering in a country where there are neither fat sausages nor cheap beer and wine is like a 3-month fast. You hardly notice how you shrink healthy. My hubby used to lose more weight in Morocco than me because my lifestyle in Europe is not much different.

Delicious recipes you'll find in the back, less with Spirulina rather exotic sharp. If you click on this book on my website www.marianne-e-meyer.com, you can read it at Amazon. But you get cosmic benefits only when you order it from your bookseller. Can you imagine why?

ISBN 978-3738609571 94 p. 17x22 cm €7,90

Please, send your completed Questionnaire to the following address:
Dr. Phil. Marianne E. Meyer
Apto. 320
P – 8801 Tavira
Or per e-mail to: DrMarianneEMeyer @ gmail.com

QUESTIONNAIRE
for the participants of the Spirulina study

Please, fill out 4-6 weeks after the daily intake of at least 10 g Spirulina
(For the purpose of the Data Protection Act your information will not be disclosed to third parties)

Name/e-mail (optional) ....

Address/phone (optional) ....

Age: .... **Gender:** (f) / (m)   **Weight:** .... kg   **Height:** .... cm

Are you smoker / non-smoker / passive smoker? (Please, underline as appropriate)

Occupation /activity: ....

Do you come into contact with chemicals, radiation, fumes or …......................…........... **?**
(Please, underline as appropriate)

How much water do you drink every day? ..... Mineral water / sparkling water / tab water
(Please, underline as appropriate)

Health problems/complaints: ....

....
Previous illnesses
....

....
1O g Spirulina (1 tbsp or 3 tsp powder or twenty 500 mg tablets) is considered a minimum daily intake preferably between meals. Since the algae expand in the stomach, it is advisable to take them with plenty of fluids, especially water, vegetable broth or juice, soup or fresh fruit juice. Alkaline liquids cleanse and detoxify. To keep detox symptoms such as nausea or diarrhea at a low level, it is recommended in the adaptation period to take the daily dose in three or more portions, starting with minimal amounts (3 x ½ or 1 tab).

1. How much Spirulina have you taken? …..

....
2. How many servings throughout the day?
....

3. Your experiences

....

....

4. What is your exercise and training program?

Please indicate which activities you perform daily (d) or weekly (w)! If weekly, how often? (..... times / w)

Hard physical work	(daily)	(...... times weekly)
Walking / Hiking	(daily)	(...... times weekly)
Swimming	(daily)	(...... times weekly)
Gymnastics	(daily)	(...... times weekly
Bicycling	(daily)	(...... times weekly)
Jogging	(daily)	(...... times weekly)
Dancing	(daily)	(...... times weekly)
Yoga	(daily)	(...... times weekly)
Other types of movement		
....	(daily)	(...... times weekly)

5. Describe your usual diet during the study, including drinks and sweets. Or write down your food of the last 3 days:

Breakfast ....

....

....

Lunch ....

....

....

Dinner ....

....

....

In-between meals …..

6. Do you take food supplements (vitamins, minerals, elixirs, herbs, etc.)? If yes, which ones?

....

....

....

7. Which drugs (legal/illegal/medically prescribed) do you take at the moment?
....

8. Which drugs/medications have you taken in the past, from an early age?
....

9. Were you able to make unusual observations while taking Spirulina?
....
....
....

10. Do you have noted any changes in:

(a Digestion	(b) Appetite	(c) Sleep	(d) Energy
(e) General condition	(f) Circulation	(g) Urine	(h) Eyes
(i) Fecal	(j) Skin/blemishes	(k) Hair	(l) Memory
(m) composition/mood	(n) susceptibility		

(o) other observed changes …...
....
....

Please, mark changes in question and explain if necessary on the back; also your other experiences during the elimination phase or anything you would like to contribute concerning your condition. Each statement is of meaning for the analysis. In the first two weeks, a variety of physical symptoms can occur. They indicate a response to the detoxification, the so-called healing crisis. Three or four times, in each case after 4 to 6 weeks, positive detox symptoms may occur such as a runny nose, scratchy throat or a cough. See the section: What reactions can occur? Also, previous illnesses can revive in short form starting with the first one.

On your way into the light, to inner freedom, serenity and always radiant health I wish you all the best!

THANK YOU FOR YOUR COOPERATION!

FOR YOUR NOTES

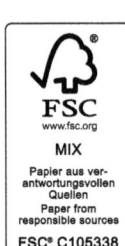